MW01612531

LIVING WITH YOUNG-ONSET PARKINSON'S DISEASE
THE FIRST FOUR YEARS

A Path Not Chosen

Notes from My Journey with a Chronic Disease

SHERRI
TOBIAS

A Path Not Chosen

NOTES FROM MY JOURNEY WITH A CHRONIC DISEASE

Sherri Tobias

MEANDERLORE PRESS

A Path Not Chosen:
Notes from my Journey with a Chronic Disease
Copyright © 2016 Sherri Tobias
First Edition (Print Version 1.4)
ALL RIGHTS RESERVED

Published by **MeanderLore Press**
P.O. Box 1222, Findlay, OH 45839

ISBN-13: 978-1-945118-00-5
ISBN-10: 1-945118-00-8

Cover Photo/Art: ©2016 Sherri Tobias
Fonts: Shadows into Light, Droid Serif

Categories:
HEA039110 HEALTH & FITNESS / Diseases / Nervous System (incl. Brain); HEALTH, FITNESS & DIETING/Diseases & Physical Ailments/ Parkinson's Disease; RELIGION & SPIRITUALITY/Spirituality/Inspirational/Health; LITERATURE/Essays & Correspondence/Diaries & Journals

Key words: Parkinson's disease, young-onset Parkinson's disease, early-onset Parkinson's disease, chronic illness, memoir, inspirational

Scripture Copyright Information
Scripture quotations marked ESV are from *The Holy Bible,* English Standard Version® (ESV®), copyright © 2001 by Crossway, a publishing ministry of Good News Publishers. Used by permission. All rights reserved.

Scripture quotations marked (NLT) are taken from the *Holy Bible,* New Living Translation, copyright © 1996, 2004, 2007 by Tyndale House Foundation. Used by permission of Tyndale House Publishers, Inc., Carol Stream, Illinois 60188. All rights reserved.

Medical Disclaimer: This book is not intended as a substitute for the medical advice of physicians. The reader should regularly consult a physician in matters relating to his/her health and particularly with respect to any symptoms that may require diagnosis or medical attention.

For the cohort that encouraged me to write

Alison, Lynne, Margie, Renee, and Shirley

Contents

Prologue

How do you react to life's detours?

~~~~~

Imagine you are zipping down a familiar highway and life is good. You left home early in order to arrive at your destination on time, but then you see a sign that thwarts all of your careful planning:

Bridge Out: Detour.

Depending on how tight your schedule is, your reactions may include a mixture of *anger, disbelief, frustration, disappointment, desperation,* and *fear.*

What started out as an enjoyable drive turns into a pop test of your character. You begin recalculating whether you will arrive late, run out of gas, get lost, or miss the event. In the process, you find that you left a few essentials at home including *humor, tranquility, patience, self-control, kindness, hope,* and *flexibility.*

When we find ourselves on a journey we did not choose, these character qualities become indispensable, yet they often elude us when we need them most.

A life detour can also wreak havoc with our plans and take us somewhere we never wanted to go, much like Dorothy in L. Frank Baum's classic, *The Wonderful*

Wizard of Oz,[1] in which she is whisked from Kansas to the Land of Oz via a cyclone.

In 2012, I started my blog, *A Path Not Chosen,* as a travelogue about the unexpected and permanent life detour I found myself on after being diagnosed with young-onset Parkinson's disease in 2011. When I decided to adapt some of the posts into a book, allusions to Baum's story were already a part of several posts I had written. Even though Baum's tale is a children's fantasy, Dorothy and her friends must face many of the very real fears we all have including natural disasters, exile, loneliness, death, enemies, failure, betrayal, purposelessness, and being lost. More parallels between my journey and the unplanned trip to Oz came to mind, so I decided to intertwine Dorothy's journey with mine.

Life detours are rarely welcome, but sometimes an unchosen path exposes us to beauty we would have missed otherwise. It can be tough to see the beautiful when we're focused on unchosen limitations, and sometimes the beauty simply isn't there to see. More often, however, we aren't prepared to see it. Only after the fact do we realized that we should have developed a better packing list or invested more time reading a guide book from someone who managed to live through the travel nightmare we face.

Whether you have yet to live through a major life detour or you are already headed down an unchosen route, this book is for you. The details of our journeys will be different, yet life's challenges evoke similar emotions

---

1 Baum, L. Frank. *The Wonderful Wizard of Oz.* Public Domain. 1900. Originally published by George M. Hill Co. (Chicago). The book was quite popular even before the annual broadcast (1959-1991) of the 1939 Metro-Goldwyn-Mayer (MGM) film adaptation, *The Wizard of Oz,* made Dorothy's journey a touchstone for more than one generation.

and responses in all of us. I would never have chosen to live with Parkinson's, but I now realize I can develop the character traits essential to finding the beauty of this new path *en route*.

Just as I found connections between my story and Dorothy's, I hope these notes help you or a loved one through some of the inevitable emotional and spiritual challenges that occur when you're journeying on a path not chosen.

Sherri Tobias
December 2015

Violet Days

May 18, 2013

~~~~~~~~

Days strung like beads upon a thread,
Black, gray, white—then black again.
Just like Dorothy without Oz
Life's in grayscale.
No breath of wind.

A wrench of heart. Ashen tears.
A levy built of cares and fears.
Senseless thoughts twist and spin.
The screen goes blank.
Pale rain begins.

But then a drop of color falls
And tendrils through the river's run.
Legion clouds cannot hold back
The caress of a long-hidden sun.

A zephyr wind begins to blow.
It dries the earth, and then we find,
Yellow roads and emerald ways
Lead us on to violet days.

Violet days come now and then
Respites from the winter's wind.
Fleeting though those days may be,
Cling tightly to the certainty
Violet days will come again.

A Storm Was Brewing

How I Landed on a Path Not Chosen

"When Dorothy stood in the doorway and looked around, she could see nothing but the great gray prairie on every side. Not a tree nor a house broke the broad sweep of flat country that reached to the edge of the sky in all directions. The sun had baked the plowed land into a gray mass, with little cracks running through it. Even the grass was not green, for the sun had burned the tops of the long blades until they were the same gray color to be seen everywhere. Once the house had been painted, but the sun blistered the paint and the rains washed it away, and now the house was as dull and gray as everything else."
~L. Frank Baum, *The Wonderful Wizard of Oz*

When our children were young and wondered why black-and-white photographs or movies lacked color, my husband would tease them and say that color didn't exist back then. It didn't take them long to call his bluff, but when I was very young, I wondered the same thing as I watched the annual televised showing of *The Wizard of Oz.*

The stark contrast between the gray world of Dorothy's home in Kansas and the Technicolor of the Land of Oz always amazed me and made me thankful I lived in a colorful world. Somehow that early lesson in being thankful for what I had faded like an old photograph over the years until I effectively became color blind. I didn't notice I had reduced my view of life to grayscale until I experienced a metaphorical cyclone that spun me onto on a path I did not choose, much like Dorothy when the twister deposited her on the Yellow Brick Road in Oz.

Early in 2011, my husband landed a job that required us to move from Pennsylvania to Ohio just a few days before my daughter finished her first year of college in Seattle. Our son said goodbye to his friends in Pennsylvania and prepared to start over at a new high school as a sophomore. After years of juggling homeschooling, volunteer roles, and part-time work, I had been exploring options and dusting off dreams that included working on my doctorate or pursuing a career. Though we all experienced the pain of leaving one path behind, the new road we traveled offered a fresh start and a trek filled with adventure and possibility.

After moving, we allowed time during the summer for vacation and visiting family. Before school started, I visited my parents. It was a pleasant visit overall, except for one seemingly minor event that will be forever etched on my memory.

On August 15, we were in the kitchen preparing a meal. My mom had taken a moment to sit down. I opened the door to the refrigerator to look for lunch options, and she asked me if I noticed my left leg was shaking.

I hadn't noticed.

It wasn't the first time my leg had been shaky, so I brushed it off. Because I exercised less consistently than I should, when I did push myself, I often had odd twitches and muscle pains. I had been trying to exercise more, and surely it was just an odd little tremor that would eventually go away.

Now I know that was the first indicator that would lead me down a path that I would never have chosen for the next part of my life's journey.

Once I was aware of the tremor, I realized it never went away when I was thinking about it. I also began having odd muscle spasms in that same leg. They were worse when I was tense or concentrating on what my leg was doing, so I chalked these symptoms up to stress and tried to ignore them.

By mid-September, pain developed in my left leg. It became severe enough that I couldn't pass it off as an exercise-related strain. The only ways I could alleviate the pain were to stand or lie on my stomach. Sitting was excruciating at times, and I became hyper-sensitive to any sort of semi-rough texture touching my legs. New to town, I didn't have a Primary Care Physician (PCP), so when I finally found one that was in my network and accepting new patients, I couldn't get an appointment until mid-October.

Because I worked from home and had not developed many outside commitments, I tried to tough it out until I could see the doctor, but it finally became too much. I headed to an urgent care clinic about ten days before my PCP appointment. After a fairly thorough examination, which included taking a set of X-rays of my spine and pelvic region, they determined that the pain was probably a result of sciatica. It was likely being caused by some sort of inflammation or disturbance in my lower spine, although the X-rays did not show any irregularities. They prescribed an anti-inflammatory medication.

The nurse practitioner also scheduled an appointment with a neurologist because she was concerned about the tremor, but it was two months in the future—a long time to wait. I went ahead and saw the PCP the following week. My pain had been alleviated by that time thanks to the medication, no exercise, and icing my lower back, so I felt a little silly going to the doctor about my odd little tremor.

Much to my surprise, the doctor didn't just laugh it off and confirm my private belief that I have hypochondriac tendencies. Instead, the tremor became the centerpiece of his examination. Besides quizzing me about my medical history, he also tested my reflexes more thoroughly than usual. I also had experienced some problems with weakness and tremors in my hands, but I attributed that to working too much on the computer.

The doctor said I needed to see a neurologist. When I said I already had an appointment, he said he would order tests to see if I needed to see the neurologist more quickly. That worried me. When he ordered blood work and a Magnetic Resonance Imaging (MRI) scan of my brain, I asked, "So what do you think is really going on?" He was noncommittal, but did not think the cause of the tremor was in my lower back. It was likely in my brain—thus the MRI. At the time, he only mentioned one disease that he wanted to rule out—multiple sclerosis (MS).

That was not what I expected.

A Storm Is Coming

The test was scheduled for the next week, so I did some research. I hadn't realized an MRI used magnetism to create the images, which was why they wanted to know if I had any metal in my body. Beyond a couple of fillings, I was safe, though I imagined more than once what it would feel like for a magnet to remove my fillings.

The MRI was less daunting than I thought it would be. I was pleased to be wearing scrubs rather than an open-backed hospital gown, and though I didn't know they were going to give me an IV to do contrast images, it wasn't so bad. I was concerned I wouldn't be able to hold my leg still enough, so I had to ask them to strap me down. They tucked a blanket around me to keep me warm, let me choose the music for my headphones, set up a mirror so I could watch what they were doing in the observation room, and slid me into the glowing tube. The music was relaxing, but when the "Oompa Loompas" who worked in the nether-regions of that glowing tomb began their jack hammering, I couldn't hear the music above the din.

Somehow I managed to lie still enough for them to get the images they needed. After going to all of that trouble (and expense), I found out a week and a half later that they'd summed up my brain in one word—unremarkable.

I still had a month to wait for my next appointment. Because the PCP gave me permission to go back to exercising and did not offer any opinions about what might really be going on, I took that as a sign that it wasn't all that dire. I didn't do much exercise beyond a few walks, and the lack of movement was taking its toll on my body. When it finally came time to see the neurologist, I had convinced myself that I was most likely wasting both his time and mine, as my pain had been virtually non-existent and the tremor, though annoying, did not interfere with my activities.

On November 30, 2011, I finally saw the neurologist. I was so positive that he would wave me out of his office and charge me double for wasting his time that I did not ask my husband to go with me to the appointment.

That would turn out to be a mistake.

The Cyclone Hits

The examination room at the neurologist's office was rather sparse. A simple wooden examination bench with a vinyl cover was the extent of the medical furnishings, aside from the obligatory patient chair, doctor's stool, and hand-washing station. When the doctor arrived, I recounted my symptoms, and he interrogated me about my family's medical history. Then we went out of the room so he could watch me walk up and down the hall. (I knew I should have practiced my runway walk before that appointment.)

After that, the neurologist did a series of tests that involved pushing and pulling with my arms and legs, reflex tests of my arms and legs, and tests to see how well I could follow moving objects with my eyes. Done with the examination, he asked me what my PCP had told me. I said he had not given me any sort of an opinion.

The neurologist must have sensed that I was frustrated about not knowing, so he came out and bluntly told me that though more testing would need to be done to rule out other diseases, he suspected some sort of Parkinsonism (a neurological disease that has Parkinson-like symptoms) if not Parkinson's disease itself.

I. Was. Floored.

Yet, all I wanted to do was laugh. An odd mixture of relief, horror, and the urge to be more positive than usual surged through me. I felt downright bubbly, and those that know me realize that is not my normal state of mind.

This was the point where I realized I should have brought my husband. I think I asked questions, but I don't remember much of the doctor's answers. He then reached up into the cabinet hanging above the sink counter and pulled out four little bottles with yellow lids. He gave me directions on how many to take and when to take them.

My response to the medication would be one way to determine if Parkinson's was the problem.

The details were a little blurry, and I think he realized that I wasn't taking everything in, as he asked me to repeat his directions back to him. He ordered another more specialized set of blood work and an MRI of my cervical spine (upper spine/neck) in order to begin ruling out other possible problems. His list was lengthier but included spinal compression, Wilson's Disease, and thyroid problems.

The strange feeling of euphoria was still present as he wrapped up the visit, and I actually made a joke of sorts, when he said I would likely have a neurologist in my life from now on. I quipped back that I hadn't really wanted to get to know him that well. But as I stood waiting for the receptionist to finish up my paper work and schedule my tests, the truth began to pop the bubbles of my odd first reactions, and I knew that I had to get out of the office before I started bawling.

I Just Want to Go Home

When I walked out of the neurologist's office, I carried an overwhelming secret. I slipped into my car and proceeded to let the pent-up tears flow, and then I had a decision to make. I could walk this new path alone, keeping the secret to myself, or I could share it, inviting others to walk along beside me.

If I chose the latter option, who would I tell? Everyone? Friends and family? Coworkers? My boss?

Because I did not expect to be diagnosed with anything serious, I had not thought about the issue—to tell or not to tell. Though my secret was more of a Pandora's box than a pleasant surprise, I still felt that irrepressible urge to share my "breaking news."

As soon as I arrived home, I told my husband. Saying I most likely had Parkinson's disease for the first time was one of the most difficult things I remember ever having to say out loud.

I don't remember what we said, but I know I cried. I know my husband held me for a long, long time. And then, I realized that I could not finish the work I had to do that evening and missed a deadline with my contractor for the first time. The events of the rest of that evening are fuzzy, but I remember a few details. My husband cooked supper. I ate supper. I spent some time curled up on my bed crying.

Like Dorothy when she landed in Oz, I wanted to go home— meaning health and the way life had been a few hours earlier when I didn't know I had an incurable disease. I don't know if after looking out the door of her relocated house into a strange land the thought crossed her mind to slam the door shut and hope by some miracle her house would be returned to its proper resting place just as quickly as it had been dislocated, but I certainly did that night.

TAKING A SECOND LOOK – CRACKING OPEN THE DOOR

Fortunately, my husband didn't let me ignore the path that lay beyond my door. Since we'd recently moved, my closest friends were not nearby. My husband suggested I write an email to a few close friends. He knew I process best through writing and that I needed the support. I managed to compose an e-mail and hit the send button.

Sending that virtual letter helped, even though my friends felt they could do nothing beyond offering prayers and what felt like insufficient words of sympathy. Neither my friends nor I realized at the time that their choice of words did not hold the power that day, it was the act of responding that contained the message I needed when I had just been excommunicated from the ranks of healthy humans. They read the opening scene of the next act in my life story that could prove to be a tragedy, and yet they wanted to know more.

In addition to my husband and the friends that I emailed, we talked to my teenage son that evening. I didn't want to worry my daughter during finals, so we waited to tell her until she came home from college the next week. A few days after that, I finally wrote my parents who were living on the other side of the world at the time. Because the diagnosis wasn't certain, for better or worse, I made the decision not to tell the rest of our family until a formal diagnosis was made. Christmas was coming, and I didn't want holiday conversations to feature Parkinson's, especially if the tests proved the neurologist's hypothesis wrong.

Plus, my emotions were simply too raw. I could write about my secret, but I wasn't sure I could say the words out loud without breaking down. It was difficult to bear that secret during the annual Christmas gathering for my husband's side of the family, but I asked my husband to wait to tell them until after New Year's once I heard back about the results of the tests. As I read books about Parkinson's in the following weeks, I learned that the decision to reveal the diagnosis of a chronic disease is a very personal matter. With young-onset Parkinson's disease, it is possible to wait years to tell people, including a spouse, depending on how quickly the external symptoms progress and how well the medications help to keep the symptoms under control.

After learning this, I began to second guess my decision to share the news so soon, yet I still felt unable to bear the weight alone. Once I started email conversations with my close friends and family I found that they wanted updates. At first I wrote personal responses but soon realized I needed to tell the same things to each person. I considered an email list, but that seemed unwieldy. Instead, I chose to create a private blog. This worked for a short time, but I soon ran into technical problems.

After some soul-searching and the realization that few people would read my blog aside from those who knew me, I made it public to simplify the process for my readers. My husband and I shared what was going on with our friends as the opportunity presented itself. We chose to let the news filter out rather than making a formal announcement to everyone we knew.

I found that as I shared my story, people responded with sympathy for my misfortune. I also found that others could empathize with me—not because they had Parkinson's disease but because they also struggled with chronic or invisible diseases or had loved ones who did. None of the interactions changed my path. No one, so far, has healed me. Yet each response was an act of love that gave me the courage to stand up, brush myself off, and start walking down a path I did not choose.

Following the Path Not Chosen

The First Year

"You must walk. It is a long journey, through a country that is sometimes pleasant and sometimes dark and terrible.... The road to the City of Emeralds is paved with yellow brick...so you cannot miss it."
~L. Frank Baum, *The Wonderful Wizard of Oz*

The first year, I had two goals: the first was to get to know my enemy and the second was to go "home" to that place of relatively good health I had enjoyed the first forty-two years of my life. Though everyone said Parkinson's had no cure, I held on to an unspoken hope that the diagnosis was wrong or that a cure would soon be discovered.

Like Dorothy and the companions she met along the way, I began following a path not chosen because I hoped I would find a way to achieve my goals if I simply moved forward and explored the new place I found myself traveling.

I started two blogs in early 2012. *A Path Not Chosen* focused on my journey with Parkinson's, while the second blog, *Walking Squared*, chronicled my choice to begin running as a way to fight the disease that may eventually rob me of my ability to move.

What follows are notes gleaned from the two blogs. Though I considered arranging the posts topically, that is not how we experience life. To better allow you to follow the ups, downs, and rabbit trails that come with any trek into undiscovered territory, I chose to leave the posts more or less in the order they were originally written.

WALKING SQUARED

January 1, 2012

Within the first two weeks after my diagnosis, I had decided to exercise and move while I could, even before I discovered that exercise and daily physical activity have been shown to alleviate Parkinson's symptoms and improve quality of life. A local women's confer-ence I sometimes attended in early March added a 5K to the weekend's activities, which gave me a goal. I downloaded a couch-to-5K plan on my phone and started running.

Two and a half weeks ago, I made a resolution—to resume exercising after a three-month hiatus. Even though the calendar did not yet read January 1, I could not wait. Health issues convinced me I could no longer lounge on the beach of inactivity.

My goal is to increase my activity level exponentially, thus I am "walking squared," which is known in modern-day English as "running." My goal for the next two months is to be able to run the square of 2.23606797749978969 64091736687313 in kilometers, which will allow me to complete my first 5K.

I am not an athlete. I never tried out for sports teams, nor did I have any desire to do so. When it comes to sports, I would be considered a "square," in the square-peg-in-a-round-hole sense of the word. As I head into 2012, however, I need a distinct goal like a 5K to help me establish this habit.

I am surprised that I now enjoy running, which I always thought of as a monotonous sport, because it enhances my thinking and mood (just like all of the athletes always claimed). So for now, this non-athlete will be attempting to walk squared for the foreseeable future, even if I never break any records or make it to the Olympics. I am in this for the fringe benefits—health and a more optimistic outlook on life.

No, I haven't gone from the couch to a marathon in two weeks, but each day I go a little farther, I am getting closer to my goal. The key is adopting the attitude of walking squared whatever your pace may be today.

Why Blog?

January 6, 2012

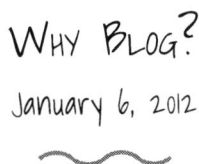

So far I am not asking, "Why me?" On the other hand, I have been wondering why I decided to share my story on a blog. After plumbing the depths of my motivations, I have come up with six reasons that hopefully prove I am not simply an exhibitionist at heart:

- **You are reading this.** For some reason, you want to know more about this new path I am headed down. Whether it is because you know me as a family member or friend, or you're trying to learn more about neurological disorders, the fact that you're reading this tells me these thoughts are important to someone.
- **I am afraid of forgetting.** I am not exactly sure why it is so crucial to remember the good, the bad, and the ugly details of life, but it is to many people, including me. Perhaps, I'll explore the reasons behind that phenomenon one day. Or, perhaps, I'll just forget.
- **I can express and explain more with the written word.** I have always been this way, and I will likely always be this way.
- **This will minimize the number of health updates I must write or share.** Talking about my new path is not taboo. So if you have a question, ask. But I do want my life to be about more than my latest ache or pain.
- **Learning about a disease can make us more sympathetic.** Even if I don't end up with as severe

or chronic a problem as the doctor now thinks, I am learning quite a bit about neurological disorders, and I will post the most interesting or relevant information here. If nothing else, this experience is beginning to make me more empathetic to those with health problems, after living forty-two years relatively illness free.

- **I am afraid of forgetting.** Oh yeah, I already covered that one.

TRAVEL UPDATE: SOME GOOD NEWS AND SOME NOT SO GOOD NEWS

January 17, 2012

~~~~~~~~

Rated PG-13. *Readers who don't like medical details cautioned. Potential violence (knife) and references to drugs.*

Let's start with the expected, yet not-so-good news. I had a follow-up visit with the neurologist yesterday to go over the results of the tests he ordered. Here are the most important questions that were answered:

Do I have Parkinson's disease?

- Yes. It is Parkinson's disease according to the neurologist's clinical diagnosis. (And no. It is not any of the other nasty Parkinsonisms mentioned.)

Did the MRI of my upper spine reveal anything?

- Yes. I have cervical spinal stenosis in my upper spine, which I should probably see a neurosurgeon about. (Just to get an opinion, mind you.) This is unrelated to the Parkinson's according to the neurologist. (Knives and spinal cord are words that should not be used in the same sentence, except to say that they should not be in the same sentence.)

Do I have to take a medication right now if I can live with the symptoms?

- No. I don't have to keep taking the medication that seems to make me happy but is also inducing insomnia. For now, I can live with the symptoms, and all the medication does is control symptoms.

- *But* yes. I should take another class of medicine that will possibly help slow down any more damage to my brain and help a little with symptoms.

Since Parkinson's is an "old person's" disease, does that mean I'm older than I think?

- No. "You are too young to have all of these problems," says the neurologist.

So does this mean I'll have to see a neurologist for the rest of my life?

- "Yes. Come see me again in four months."

Though I'm glad to have answers, I now have another list of questions:

- Do I seek another opinion about the Parkinson's diagnosis?
- Do I go see the neurosurgeon and open up another Pandora's Box?
- Do I take the medication that may or may not help?
- Beyond my self-prescribed exercise therapy that I have already started, do I explore other options beyond traditional medicine?

Fortunately, I have some good news to report:

- My first day of teaching went well.
- It is raining buckets rather than snowing heaps. (Though those by the river that sometimes floods may not agree that this is good.)
- Despite the dreary time of year and circumstances, I haven't been dealing with depression like I often do in the winter.
- My 5K training is progressing.

Yes, despite the not-so-good news, I have much to be thankful for.

No Whine (or Wine) Allowed

January 23, 2012

Though I was tempted to start this out with a sip of w[h]ine, I am afraid it has been removed from the list of my allowable comestibles. Instead, I'll start out with a quote from James, who seems bent on making a teetotaler out of my mind:

Count it all joy, my brothers, when you meet trials of various kinds. ~ James 1:2, ESV

I don't know if James was thinking of physical and psychological difficulties when he mentions "various trials," but that is what is on my plate at the moment. So far, whether it is the blessing of being in denial or simply a God-given peace about this new path, I have had more joy in the past few weeks than not. (And then again, I have had a few of those "hit-the-wall" moments, as well.)

It is what may not be on my plate and in my cup (as of yesterday) that is tempting me to descend into the anti-joyful habit of whining. My new medication requires me to avoid quite a number of foods. Most (like caviar, fermented bean curd, Spam, aged meats, and alcohol) are not problematic, as they aren't part of my usual diet, but when basics like aged cheeses, spinach, bananas, chocolate, and homemade bread are on the list, then that siren of whining begins to wail within me, "Don't tell me what I can't eat!"

I am one hundred percent certain my family noticed my whining the past couple of days, since I have been doing research and printing out lists of everything I can't eat.

Then James came uninvited to my pity party reminding me to count it all joy.

- I have a medication that may help me.
- I have the means to get medical care.
- Many foods remain on my "can eat" list.

And those are just the rather self-absorbed joys that popped into my head first.

I know I am still in the early stages of processing this change, but if I have learned anything from my research, I know it is beneficial to have a positive attitude. So, here's hoping I can keep counting it all joy by focusing on the "cans" rather than the "cannots," and by permanently eliminating whine from my diet.

So How Are You Feeling?

February 8, 2012

~~~~~~~~

I am not sorry I let people know about my diagnosis of Parkinson's disease, and it is gratifying that so many ask how I am doing. Despite this, I find it is hard to answer the simple question, "So how are you feeling?"

After the crisis of being diagnosed, life is surprisingly better and busier than it had been. My family finally seems to be settling in to our new hometown, I enjoy being back in the classroom, I am running three to five times a week, and I am happier than I have been in a long time.

Physically, my symptoms are about the same as they have been since this all began. I am not allowing them to interfere with much of life. Sure, some days are better than others, but that's the way it is with even the healthiest person. In some ways, I feel a bit like the boy who cried wolf.

It is not easy for people to know what to do with a chronic, degenerative disease. After the initial shock, you find the fire brigade needs sent home without quenching the flames because it can't be done.

Being diagnosed with Parkinson's is a bit like finding out you are living on an island that is not as solid as you originally thought. It is floating on molten lava, a simmering fire that is too vast for mortals to subdue. At first, this realization is terrifying, but then you realize that you've been living on this island all your life. And so, you continue on with a greater respect for what lies beneath your feet.

So for today, that's how I am feeling.

Acceptance or Change?

February 29, 2012

~~~~~~

I don't usually publish a post until I have thought through the content and come to a conclusion, but I am going to take a risk and post a thought that is still in process.

This past Sunday, I had one of those "the pastor's been reading my mind" moments, even though I know pastors do not consider clairvoyance a spiritual gift. Here's the snippet of Ephesians 4:1 (NLT) that tipped me off:

Therefore I, a prisoner for the Lord....

Yes. That is it. The subject of the sermon was unity in the church, but that is not what I have been thinking about. I have not even been contemplating imprisonment or Paul, for that matter.

If you even take the time to notice that phrase before leaping into the rest of the passage, the first question that comes to mind is why Paul slipped that tidbit in before he tackled the subject of Christian unity. While this is a good question, what caught my attention was another question that was raised:

Why was Paul writing a letter of exhortation to a church while he was a prisoner?

If any of us ended up in prison, we'd more likely spend time studying the law and writing letters so that we could get out of prison than simply accepting our role as a prisoner and sending encouraging epistles to those outside our prison's walls. And that is what meshed with the thought that is still in process.

Lately, I have been reading up on neuroscience and the brain because that is where Parkinson's disease begins. Much is being learned, and our understanding of the brain is changing in radical ways. Much effort is being poured into finding ways to cure neurological disorders like Parkinson's and Alzheimer's disease, and my interest level in these topics has increased ten-fold thanks to my diagnosis.

Though general biology was never a subject of interest for me, neuroscience is intriguing because the study of the brain intersects with the mind, and dare I say the soul—the essence of who we are as humans.

The more I read about the brain and health in general, the more often I have the unsettling feeling we're chasing the ghost of Juan Ponce de León in his quest to find the Fountain of Youth. Our questions give us away:

- How can we live longer?
- How can we eat to be healthier?
- What activities should we do to be stronger?
- How can we have a better quality of life?

Make no mistake, I dislike being ill just as much as the next person. If I could choose a life path, it would not include a degenerative disease. But Paul's acceptance of being a prisoner while maintaining his outward focus makes me pause and ponder other questions, which I either do not have answers for or the answers are unsettling. (Remember, this is a thought in process.)

- To what extent should we strive to prolong or enrich our earthly lives?
- How can we know when to accept the unchangeable or to fight for that which should be changed?
- Why do we celebrate physical healing?
- What about all of the people who are not healed?

- And finally, are we looking for the Fountain of Youth in all the wrong places?

Yes, I am ending with more questions than answers, but I warned you that this was a thought still in process.

The Difference a Day and a Pill Make

March 7, 2012

~~~~~~

About a week and a half ago, I'd had it. I hate taking medication. I hate supplements. I didn't like the dietary changes I was making because of a new medication that didn't seem to be doing any good. Then again, I kept forgetting to take the second dose of the new medication most days. Since I had already tapered off my medication due to my forgetfulness, I simply stopped taking it. And no, I did not consult my doctor.[1]

Over the week and a half I was off medication, I began noticing subtle changes. I got tired earlier in the afternoon, and in the evening about all I could do was curl up on the couch and vegetate. When I ran, I had more problems with muscle fatigue and foot cramps. My mood went downhill.

Monday night I slept restlessly, never able to get comfortable. Tuesday morning, I awoke feeling the worst I had in a long time, and I realized that I needed to break my medication fast. Tuesday was still a bit of a blur, but I rested well last night. This morning, it is like I am a different person.

I would chalk up sixty to seventy percent of the difference to a good night's sleep. The rest lies in the pill, but not in the way you might think.

It is unlikely, given the nature of Parkinson's medications, that one dose made that much difference. The medications tend to be more effective as you take them over a period of time. It is what taking that pill signifies

---

1 I do not recommend making changes to your medication without consulting your doctor.

mentally and emotionally that may have made the difference. Popping that pill in my mouth was a surrender and signified that I was accepting some issues that I have been wrestling with for a while.

I have Parkinson's, and it affects me more than I have wanted to admit. In my research I discovered that Parkinson's symptoms can get worse immediately after discontinuing a medication, which may be what I experienced this past week. Even though it is possible I could have toughed it out and my body would have regulated itself in time, this experience taught me I do have Parkinson's symptoms and many are subtler than my leg and hand tremors. Much of what I thought was due to aging or working out too hard is likely caused or exacerbated by the Parkinson's, including odd aches and pains, overly sensitive skin, fatigue, and depression. It is even possible that my decreased sense of smell, which began over ten years ago, could have been a precursor or indicator that I would develop Parkinson's.

I need medications to help me alleviate symptoms if I want to function as well as I can. It is a tough thing to accept that my brain isn't working properly, and I will likely be taking one medication or another for the rest of my life. (Unless, of course, they find a way to reverse or cure the disease within my lifetime.)

It is also tough to admit that it takes medication to keep my brain from descending into negativity or depression. I have struggled against this for over ten years, trying to retrain my thought patterns so that I would not have to take medications to control my depressive tendencies. It feels a bit like giving in to defeat to admit that the Parkinson's medications help my depression, but that is the one symptom that is the most crucial to regulate as it is easier to deal with physical symptoms if I am emotionally and mentally healthy.

And finally, I don't like being told what I can and cannot eat. The main reason I have rebelled against my current medication is that I don't like the dietary restrictions that are recommended to prevent hypertensive side effects. Further research and a talk with my pharmacist seem to indicate that I do not have to follow the restrictive diet at the dosages I am taking, which has relieved that area of stress. But I hope that if I need to give up certain foods in the future, I can accept the change more gracefully than I did this time.

What a difference a day (and a pill) can make.

LIFE-A-THON

March 10, 2012

~~~~~

I met a New Year's (okay, more like Advent) resolution for the first time. I trained and completed a 5K. I couldn't run the whole way, but I did finish. In fact, for my age group, I came in first. Granted it was a small race and many participants walked, but it was a satisfying way to wrap up this grand exercise experiment.

So what's next?

Maybe, I could do another 5K or step it up and see if I can make my body do a 10K. Then, there are half marathons and marathons and triathlons. And then again, maybe not. I began exercising not to compete but to live a better life. The 5K gave me a short-term goal to strive for.

One thing I learned from the process is that exercise is more of a psychological battle than a physiological one. Sure, you have to push your body, but it is the mind that holds the carrot on the stick. If I gave myself small goals within a longer run, it was much easier than staring at that long stretch as a whole. When I wanted to give up, I would challenge myself to do thirty more seconds or one more block. When I got there, I'd ask myself if I could do it again. Those short goals added up to longer and longer runs over time.

Exercise is essential when fighting Parkinson's. I can't quit now. On December 25, 2011, I began training for a life-a-thon. The distance is daunting, so I won't look that far ahead. Instead, I plan to challenge myself to exercise just one more day, and when I've done that I'll ask myself to do it again.

PLEASE, DON'T CALL ME "THAT PARKINSON'S WOMAN"

April 21, 2012

ike a caricature artist, we often exaggerate a single trait or feature of people we know, and in our minds, they are forever associated with that one trait. Maybe she's "the woman with big hair" twenty-five years after the style ceased to be fashionable. Or maybe he is "the complainer" or "the class clown."

When a person is first afflicted with a chronic disease, it shoves its way through the crowd, claiming attention like a spoiled diva. Knowing about the disease, fighting the disease, and learning to cope with a chronic disease can consume a patient during the first few months, and eventually, we may find it difficult to separate the person from the disease. In our mind, she has become the "fibromyalgia woman," or he has become the "man with Alzheimer's." Yet a person is so much more than a disease.

After choosing to share my challenge with Parkinson's, my health became one of the first topics of conversation whenever I would see some people, especially if we didn't see each other frequently. I began to regret having shared the news in some cases because I felt I was coming to be seen as "that Parkinson's lady," and I didn't like it. The post, "The Blind Man, the Leper, and the Paralytic," was my response.

THE BLIND MAN, THE LEPER, AND THE PARALYTIC

*O*nce upon a time, a long time ago, there lived a blind man, a leper, and a paralytic. As it happened, each one of them lived in the same country at the same time, and it just happened to be a blessed time, despite the political turbulence in that land.

It was a blessed time because a miracle man walked the earth then. He had the power to make the blind man see, to cleanse the leper, and to loose the paralytic's frozen limbs. And as happens in tales that begin with "once upon a time," there was a happy ending for these three, as the miracle man used his healing powers to rid each one of them of their physical limitations. He rubbed spit and dirt on the blind man's eyes, and he could see again. He had pity on the leper (and his nine friends), and they were cleansed. He forgave the paralytic's sins, and he could walk again.

Despite the good fortune of these three, the storytellers did not write down the men's names, and now we only know them by their disabilities, even though they were healed.

This is a bit unsettling to me, since I don't want to be identified as "the Parkinson's woman." I could have kept it a secret to avoid this title, but it is too late. My family knows, and the news has been filtering out to other friends and acquaintances, as well. And hey, I started a blog about it, so if everyone happened onto my site, technically, the whole world could know, though I am doubtful that would ever happen.

So what I am grappling with now is not whether people know about my challenge so much as whether I am being defined by it. While I want to be knowledgeable about what I may face and how I can slow down its pro-gression or alleviate the symptoms, it is important to me that the focus of my life is not this disease—even if down the road it increases my physical limitations and neces-sarily becomes a more central part of my daily existence. While I am indebted to those who work tirelessly to find a cure, after much consideration I do not think that my path leads in the direction of research or fundraising given my gifts and abilities.

So if I will never become a research scientist searching for the cure nor a fund-raising advocate, am I ungrateful and fatalistic? Am I giving in when I should be fighting harder?

Even more hard-hitting: do I lack faith if I accept that I may live with this condition the rest of my life, not seek-ing or expecting healing?

I don't know the answers to those questions, so for now, they'll remain questions without answers. What I do know is that for every person who has been physically healed by the miracle man, there are a dozen or maybe hundreds and thousands that have not been given the relief of physical healing in this lifetime. But whether we're healed or not healed, everyone has one thing in common—we all must live during the time we're given.

So, I think again about the blind man, the leper, and the paralytic. The blind man is known because he was the blind man who could see. The leper is known because he was the leper who was cleansed. The paralytic is known because he was the paralytic who walked. More impor-tantly, we know their stories because they encountered a man of miracles, who is the protagonist of the story after all. He knew their names then, and he knows their names now, even if we never will.

These three people had limitations that defined who they were. Based on the way he healed the paralytic by forgiving him, it is clear that the healing went beyond a mere rearrangement of the person's cells. The miracle man helped each of them overcome their defining limitation so they could live more fully. I may or may not ever be healed of Parkinson's, but if I must be known as "that Parkinson's woman" then I hope I can be that Parkinson's woman who lived a full life.

Avoided the Knife

May 3, 2012

~~~

Today I finally saw a neurosurgeon about the spinal stenosis that was discovered during one of the MRIs I had during the diagnosis phase, and I now know the relief that the knife thrower's assistant must feel when she has managed to avoid the knives.

The neurosurgeon had no revelations. This time, the results of the consult were as I expected. He concurred with the neurologist that my symptoms are more likely caused by Parkinson's disease than spinal stenosis. After a talk, a look at my MRIs, and a brief examination, he said that recommending surgery at this point would only be for his benefit, not mine, and he has plenty to do without manufacturing unneeded surgeries. (Yes, a neurosurgeon with a sense of humor.)

After talking about the stenosis and showing on the MRI why it would not require surgery at this point, he pulled up the MRI scans of my brain. Then, he proceeded to take me on a tour of my brain just for the fun of it. I couldn't wrap my mind around the fact I was looking at pictures of my brain. What creeped me out the most was when he scrolled down far enough into the layers of images to expose my eyeballs. The image confirmed that the term "eyeball" is an accurate description. He also scored points when he declared that I was young and skinny.

This is the first medical exam I've experienced where God was mentioned at least three times by the physician, and he didn't know us or our religious persuasion. The references just seemed to flow naturally from his lips with no artifice or pretension. He mentioned having to give a patient the bad news that he didn't just have a spinal problem but also had a debilitating disease with a short life expectancy. The surgeon said God doesn't usually make people deal with two major health problems, but in some cases he does. Food for thought.

I am glad that for now I have avoided the neurosurgeon's knife. For a doctor's visit, it was quite enjoyable.

Going on Six Months: A Travel Update

May 18, 2012

~~~~

It has been about six months since I was told I had Parkinson's disease. It is hard to believe it has been that long. My condition is stable, as far as I can tell, with the main symptoms being the tremors in my left arm and leg as well as some muscle stiffness. I have some days where I am fatigued for no reason, but exercising definitely helps all of my general symptoms except for the tremor.

Today, I had a follow-up appointment. My neurologist took me off the medication I have been taking because it is not helping my symptoms. So, he is having me try a new one. He said if it works, my tremors should get better, although they most likely won't go away completely. He also said it should help the dystonia (involuntary muscle contractions) in my left foot and toes when I run. It is the same class of medication as the first one I tried. It caused insomnia, so we'll see how this goes.

The Need to Create

May 21, 2012

~~~~~~~~

My need to create has increased since my diagnosis. I don't know if this is because a medical condition reminds us of our mortality or if the medications are changing my brain's chemistry. Maybe it is a little of both.

Whatever the case, I finally finished a cookbook project I started years ago. I realize it already needs to be updated and is a bit archaic when the Internet is our recipe book, but it was good to finish the first version of that project.

In February, I finally began a creative sewing project that I had thought about for a number of years. Since the sewing is all by hand, part of my motivation was to take on a project that exercises my fine motor skills. It also gives me something productive to do when we watch movies or television shows.

Now that I am on summer break from teaching, I am dusting off some of my writing projects and considering new ones. I am also taking the time to learn how to better use the Adobe Creative Suite software that has been sitting on my computer since I took web design courses almost two years ago. How these two activities will merge has yet to be determined, but maybe I'll be able to complete a short project or two this summer.

Here's hoping I have the stamina and perseverance to see some of these things through to completion.

KEEP AT IT (EXERCISE THAT IS)
May 27, 2012

*B*eing persistent when it comes to exercise is tough, isn't it? Over the years, I have been a "seasonal exerciser." After the eating season (which is autumn for me), I would be motivated to move long enough to rid myself of the excess weight during the exercise season (winter/spring). Summer was a toss-up, depending on how hot it was and how slowly the weight came off during the exercise season.

Then when I found that exercise was an important part of my treatment for Parkinson's disease, I decided I wanted to take up running. (Don't ask me why.) Fortunately, this fell in line with my usual pattern of notching up my exercise routine following the Christmas holidays.

I have been doing fairly well at running since Christmas, but Parkinson's has literally cramped my style. After about ten to twenty minutes of running, that pesky dystonia I have in my left foot makes it curl up inside my shoe. It's rather like trying to run with hoof instead of a foot, or so I imagine. In the past, this would have torpedoed my exercise routine, but I knew I couldn't let that happen this time.

I still don't like the thought of exercising, but I have learned a few ways to "keep at it" over the last few months.

- **There's nothing like an outside motivator to keep you moving.** It doesn't need to be as drastic as being diagnosed with a chronic disease, though that has definitely helped me dig deep and make time for activity. Deciding to run the 5K in March gave me a short-term goal that helped me persist even when my foot cramps made me want to stop.

- **Don't look too far down the road.** If you are not a natural-born exerciser, don't think about the fact that you should exercise for the rest of your life. Don't sit down and calculate out how many hours of your life you will spend on exercise if you start now. Instead, take it one day at a time and focus on what you can do today.

- **On the other hand, do commit to make exercise a part of your routine.** Each morning I think about how I can work physical activity into my schedule. Some days it is an early morning run. Other days, exercise has to wait for an after-dinner walk with my husband. When it is too hot, cold, or rainy, I pop in an exercise DVD or use the treadmill. I am currently exploring whether I can outfit my bike with baskets or panniers so I can use it to run errands for exercise with a purpose.

- **Be realistic, but also challenge yourself.** I was disappointed when I realized I would most likely have to walk some of the 5K in March, but I decided to go through with it anyway. I did have to take walking breaks, but as soon as my foot was ready, I went back to jogging. Some days, I don't have the energy to do a full-blown workout, so I do something gentler like Pilates or yoga or a simple walk around the block. On the days I feel good, I try to go a little faster or a little further to give my body a challenge.

- **Celebrate milestones.** I don't spend a lot of time tracking my exercise beyond trying not to go more than one day without intentional activity. I do, however, clip on my iPod Nano and use Nike+ to record my distance and time any time I walk or run. The data is automatically recorded for me whenever

I sync my iPod. I check in every week or so to see how I am doing. It is gratifying to see the kilometers stack up.

I am going to take this opportunity to put the last tip into practice. After taking a new medication for about a week, I already have two victories to celebrate:

- I beat my race-day 5K time.
- I ran twenty-five minutes without my foot cramping.

Today, I am taking a break for my birthday, but tomorrow, I'll be back out there keeping at it.

STEPPING OUT

May 30, 2012

〜〜〜

According to several resources that I read in my initial research binge, it is important for those with Parkinson's disease to avoid withdrawing from social interaction. Those dealing with Parkinson's may want to avoid being with people for a number of reasons:

- They may have embarrassing external symptoms like a severe tremor, dyskinesia (involuntary tics or movements), freezing, or drooling.
- Depression (which often accompanies Parkinson's) reduces their desire to interact with others.
- Stress often exacerbates the symptoms of Parkinson's, so avoiding stressful situations becomes a strategy that may lead to withdrawal from social activities.

At this point, my external symptoms are mild, so the first excuse doesn't explain my reticence about stepping out and getting involved in things away from home.

The last two reasons, however, have affected my decisions about social interaction for more than ten years, which is one reason why I believe the Parkinson's began several years before it was diagnosed. This year, I have made changes that have helped me step out and get more involved in the community.

- In January, I started a new job after working online for six years. I am back to teaching English to Speakers of Other Languages (ESOL) at a nearby university. Interacting with the students and my coworkers has been beneficial.

- Soon after going back to work, I began a two-year-long leadership training program sponsored by my denomination. This is stretching me as I have never seen myself as a leader.
- Beginning this blog was another step out of my comfort zone, which has unexpectedly opened up some opportunities to talk with people about Parkinson's.
- Instead of writing at my dining room table, I chose to ride my bike downtown to write at a coffee shop, where I sometimes run into people I know.

I may have to make the last activity a habit. As long as I bike or walk to the coffee shop, I may be able to justify a frozen chai latte with whipped cream every now and again. Here's to stepping out!

The Number of Our Days

June 11, 2012

~~~~~~~~

It is summer and thousands are flocking to the beach to carefully spend one precious week of vacation. We determine to enjoy every moment, yet we can never quite forget our time is ticking down and our brief week in paradise will come to an end. Few would compare life to a vacation, yet many of us view death with a dread that is not so far removed from the feelings that we have about the inevitable conclusion of a dream getaway.

The other day while I was running, a song by Christine Denté popped up in the play list I had chosen. I had heard the song many times but never truly listened to its message before that moment. A line from the song "Good-Bye," caused me to consider a shift in the way I think of life and death.

After an opening verse that sets the stage—someone has died—Denté considers the response of those left behind. In the chorus, she encourages us not to worry about death because "we need not stay longer than the number of our days."[1]

I have often questioned why Christians mourn death since we have the hope of a better life when we slip beyond this world. Not only do we mourn for those who have died, but many of us fear our own death and do what we can to prolong life on earth. Is this because life is so good here, or is our faith in life after death less certain than we say it is? If earth is the vacation followed by a dark unknown, it makes sense to dread death; however, after

---

1 Dente, Christine. "Good-Bye," *Becoming*. Rocketown Records, 2003.

truly hearing the line in "Good-Bye" for the first time, I wonder if our view of life on earth is the true source of our fear and worry.

To say that we *need not stay longer* on earth reverses the metaphor. While there is a purpose for our time here, shouldn't we have a healthy longing for heaven in much the same way we look forward to a vacation?

Though the separation of death causes pain and loss, perhaps, the limitations we live under on earth make us short-sighted. If our loved ones go on vacation and leave us behind, we miss them, but we also wish them well (once we get past our jealousy at their good fortune of heading to the beach without us). Isn't this how we should view the death of those who die in Christ?

Reversing the metaphor also changes the countdown to one of anticipation. Knowing our days are numbered should assure us that our life on earth is never too short or too long, though we may not understand the ways or the wisdom of God in these matters.

Please understand I am not saying that overcoming the fear of death is as easy as flipping around the words in a sentence or that we should not grieve for those we lose. On the contrary, Christ has offered us hope especially when we fear death or mourn for those who have died. I am also not recommending that we take the end of our life into our own hands when we don't feel like life is worth living. It is God that knows the number of our days, not us.

Jesus promised his disciples he would be going ahead to prepare a place for them in his Father's house. I imagine it will surpass any beach-front property we've experienced yet. We can be assured that the bills have already been paid and the reservations made. Though we can't put the exact date on our calendars, we can rest in the fact that we need not put off our departure longer than the number of our days.

ONLY THE PHYSICIANS

June 13, 2012

~~~~~~

When you buy a white car, you notice how many other people own white cars (especially when you forget where you parked at the local mall). When you're pregnant, every other woman you see is pregnant, and you make inane comments about the water supply causing an epidemic of mothers-to-be. Yet nothing has changed but your perspective.

About seven months ago, my perspectives on health began to change. I had always considered myself a relatively healthy person, and when you have health, you don't think about it. You may not even realize what you have until you lose it. Then, it becomes like the pearl of great price you will do anything to attain.

During the seven months since my diagnosis, I have been hunting for that pearl. I have read books, scoured the Internet, and seen doctors. While many research projects show great promise, none have cracked the code and revealed a cure for Parkinson's disease.

So I find myself in a holding pattern when it comes to learning more about the disease. Like an airplane pilot waiting for the signal to land, I am going in circles. Each book or article I read comes back to the same conclusions:

- Parkinson's is an incurable disease.
- The symptoms can be treated, but not indefinitely.
- Many of the ongoing research studies show promise, but none have found the "magic bean" that will cure

the seven to ten million people who struggle with this disease worldwide.[1]

These are not the answers I want when it comes to my search for renewed health.

This morning I was reading II Chronicles, one of the historical books in the Old Testament of the Bible. The writer was giving an overview of the reign of King Asa, the third king of Judah, and the story ended like this:

> *In the thirty-ninth year of his reign, Asa developed a serious foot disease. Yet even with the severity of his disease, he did not seek the Lord's help but turned only to his physicians.[2]*

In the past, I most likely would have skimmed right over this sentence, but because my perspective on healing and health has changed, it caught my attention. With a two-sentence limit on wrapping up Asa's life, why did the writer point out that Asa only consulted physicians about a physical condition that may have brought about the end of his life two years later?

For the most part, Asa had been a good king, but he had sought help from a neighboring nation rather than divine help when faced with a war with the northern kingdom of Israel. A prophet admonished him for not seeking and trusting in God's help. The scripture says Asa was angry with the prophet, but I have to imagine he was really angry with God, the source of the admonishment. Given Asa's unwillingness to seek God about his foot, the anger and distrust apparently continued during the few short years he had left.

1"Statistics on Parkinson's." *Parkinson's Disease Foundation.* 2015. Web.
2 II Chronicles 13:12, NLT

After some thought, I realized I have been spending so much time consulting only the "physicians" that I have ignored the One who is the source of healing. But why? Underneath it all, am I angry with God about the Parkinson's? Or do I not trust that God will heal me?

While I believe he is the source of healing, not everyone who seeks him is healed. I have to wonder whether God would have healed Asa's foot if he had sought God, and if he had not been healed, could he have trusted that God's decision was best? Can I?

THE STRENGTH OF LIMITATIONS

June 15, 2012

~~~~~~

Though we begin life as infants limited by our physical size, lack of knowledge, and life experience, one by one, we take on the challenges presented by those limitations, which paradoxically help us to grow in strength, knowledge, and wisdom.

When we reach our teen years or early adulthood, we've overcome enough of our limitations that we begin to see life as a buffet of options that stretches beyond the visible horizon. The number of choices both excites and sometimes paralyzes us.

If the chef suggests where we should start, we are freed to eat because of limitation. His suggestion reduces our options to one, yet we don't tend to see the freedom that limitation offers us. Some say they are not restricted by limitations and try to prove it by ignoring the chef's suggestions and choosing a different course to begin their meal. Yet by embracing their freedom, they have self-limited themselves to the untried dishes on the buffet. Those who take the chef's suggestion accept limitation in the guise of opportunity and invitation because it allows them to act when they don't know where to start.

When we are young, we believe that any part of the buffet is still available to us no matter where we choose to start. If we get tired of one type of food, we can move to another. We can be whatever we want to be in the buffet of life from a connoisseur of sushi to a fast-food aficionado.

At some point, however, we will find that a drought or other major event has caused a key ingredient to become difficult or impossible to procure. If a civil war or epidemic shuts down the world's largest producer of cacao beans, the all-chocolate table in the dessert section would no longer be an option. We can do little to nothing about large-scale limitations except to embrace them as we did when we were infants and children and see how they help us to grow.

So far Parkinson's only affects my potential future, but I know my choices in life's buffet will become limited sooner rather than later without breakthroughs in understanding and treating the disease. While I am working to delay that outcome, I am also considering how I will react to a more limited life. Will I look at all that I could consume and despair that my stomach is not big enough or my time is not long enough to eat it all? Or will I be satiated with the sustenance that lies within my grasp?

Perhaps, we need to think back to our beginning when limitations were imposed on us as infants and children and we did not even know it. We know from experience that limitation can break us if we give up, but it can also help us to act with greater creativity, purpose, and precision if we allow limitation to strengthen us.

When and if the time comes that I am unable to communicate with my body, I can only hope that God gives me the ability to develop new strengths within a new set of limitations.

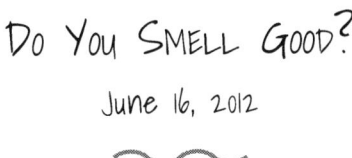

Do You Smell Good?

June 16, 2012

I have an old and overdone joke I pull out when I don't notice an unpleasant odor that everyone else does—

I don't smell so good.

What I really mean, however, is that I don't smell well, as my sense of smell has been on the fritz for over a decade.

I used to be hypersensitive to scents, and I am still almost overcome by dizziness when I enter Bath and Body Works stores. On the other hand, I don't detect other smells. This is disappointing when I can't smell baking cinnamon rolls or a flower, but it is also a perk. I don't usually notice when a skunk has perfumed the neighborhood or the farmers are fertilizing the fields.

Up until my Parkinson's diagnosis, I chalked this symptom up to the many allergies I either developed or discovered as a young adult. There is growing evidence, however, that hyposmia (a reduced ability to detect scents), may be one of the earliest symptoms of Parkinson's. Another piece of the Parkinson's mystery may have been sniffed out.

SPILLING OUT

July 3, 2012

~~~~~

W e were in the path of the *derecho* (land hurricane) that plowed across the eastern U.S. last Friday. Our power went out as soon as the winds started, and we're still waiting for that magical moment when the lights go on again. It could be another four to five days before ninety percent of our local power is restored.

This is one of those "glass jostling" events when whatever is in the glass spills out. So far most people have resigned themselves to the wait, but then there are those moments when the frustration, impatience, and anger at this unexpected change bubbles up and spews out. Thankfully, there are also many who are filled with the gifts of grace, service, and generosity, all of which help to wash away the more poisonous reactions to this forced lifestyle change.

Even though this is a temporary change, it has been a reminder to keep the reservoirs of my heart and mind filled with contents that I don't mind others seeing, because when glass-jostling events come, whatever is inside will spill out.

The Two Sides of Transparency

July 10, 2012

~~~~~~

Once someone is transparent about a difficult issue, it not only puts them in a vulnerable position, but it imposes that vulnerability on anyone who relates to them. Sometimes it is easier not to know, isn't it?

The article, "Keeping Parkinson's a Secret"[1] in yesterday's *New York Times*, reveals the difficulty of making the decision to be transparent about Parkinson's. For those living with Parkinson's, keeping the secret can increase stress. Secrets require us to screen what we say and make excuses for physical symptoms. For some, the burden becomes too much, and they decide to shine a light on their condition and tell others about their health challenge.

For the person with the disease, it is natural to focus on the difficulties, but what about the person who is on the outside peering in?

If you learn someone you love or are acquainted with has a chronic condition, it can make you feel helpless or awkward. You want to do something, but you don't know what. Do you say anything or keep quiet? Do you avoid the person or spend more time with them? Do you mention the disease or pretend it doesn't exist? If you can't honestly say you know what they are going through, sometimes it feels safer to turn your back altogether to avoid being exposed to the issues revealed by transparency.

Now that I am on the inside of the screen door, I have had to deal with other people's reactions to my news. I am

---

1 Yandell, Kate. "Keeping Parkinson's a Secret," *New York Times*, 9 Jul 2012.

discovering we often react to chronic illnesses in much the same way we do death—even if the disease is not communicable or immediately life threatening. We fear it. We shun it. We feel inadequate in the face of something so much bigger than ourselves.

The examples in the *New York Times* article reveal that people diagnosed with Parkinson's have different reasons for hiding their condition. Some patients don't want the attention it will bring, or they don't want to worry or bother others. Some are in denial. Others are concerned the revelation could cost them their job or other freedoms.

When a friend does reveal her situation to you, she may put conditions on what you can and cannot share. Though this may be difficult, be sensitive to her wishes. (Use discernment if what she asks could put your friend or others at risk, however.)

Here are a few ways friends and family can respond helpfully to transparency:

- **Avoid dwelling on the illness, but do talk about it.** If it comes up in conversation, it is okay. If an issue needs addressed, bring it up. This is a part of life now, but it is not *all* of life.

- **Treat your friend, co-worker, or acquaintance the same as you did the day before the screen became transparent (unless, of course, you treated her badly in the first place).** She is the same person, even if she now has an undesirable and ever-constant companion in tow. No, you can't understand exactly what she is going through, so focus on being the supportive family member, friend, or co-worker you always have been.

- **Look for ways to challenge and empower the person physically, emotionally, and mentally.** Yes, it is good to help, but it is also important not to send your friend to the nursing home prematurely. Parkinson's (especially young-onset Parkinson's) can progress very slowly. Though I am not a medical doctor, from what I have read it makes much more sense for those with Parkinson's to continue to do as many of their usual activities as possible for as long as they can. New challenges may also be beneficial to keeping the mind, body, and soul fit.

- **Steer conversations away from complaints and pessimism when you can.** Depression is a common side effect or companion to many long-term illnesses, Parkinson's included. Constantly dwelling on the negatives can make this worse. I have dealt with depression off and on for many years. I don't like it when a brave soul points out that I am more pessimistic than usual or that my complaint meter is in the red zone, but I need to hear it. Over the years, I have become more adept at monitoring this myself, but I still have days when I give Eeyore, Puddleglum, and Marvin, the Paranoid Android (pick your genre) a run for their money.

- **Share information you learn about the disease, but leave it at that.** I appreciate friends who think of me when they hear about a potential therapy. If it is something new to me, I usually investigate it, but I am in the process of working with my doctors and doing my own research, so it may or may not be the right option for me. Because Parkinson's manifests its symptoms differently in each patient and has no cure, experimentation and theories of treatment options abound. Discerning which are valid options and which are quackery and magic beans can be difficult in those first months. So share, but don't push.

It can be tough when the light comes on and a friend reveals her new challenge. Instead of staring through the screen door wondering what you can do, open it. By letting you know what she is facing, your friend has invited you inside.

Your Mind: Don't Go on Vacation Without It

July 24, 2012

~~~~~~

t is the time of year when vacations are in full bloom. People are crisscrossing the country on their way to the perfect location to get away from it all. But others are experiencing a vacation drought for one reason or another. They can't afford it. They can't take the time off. Or they simply want a vacation from something that is impossible to leave at home—like a chronic illness.

It is interesting that the ideal vacation is at least a week long at a location several hours or more from home. That is not always possible, so we've developed vacation hybrids like the long weekend, the mini-vacation, the day trip, and the stay-cation.

I think there is something to this. While a multi-week pilgrimage to the beach, mountains, or a fascinating city can help some relax and rejuvenate, most of us have experienced a vacation where the cares of normal life hopped in the car on the way out the driveway and became an annoying backseat driver the whole way there and back. Upon pulling up to the house on your return, you realize that you might as well have stayed at home. And in a sense, you did. Your body may have traveled hundreds of miles, but your mind stayed home.

We spend hours planning a trip, working to pay for it, making our packing lists and checking them twice. We may spend days moving our physical selves to an alternative location and back again. Yet, we often overlook the intangible in our frenzy—our minds and our souls need to be prepared for the Sabbath that a vacation represents. We need to be prepared for the new perspective offered by a change of pace, activity, or location. We need to allow time to step back from the cares of life and focus on other things for a time.

Maybe a trip to the beach or the city isn't possible for you this year. That's okay. You can give yourself a mind and soul vacation by changing your routine. Head out to a new coffee shop tomorrow morning, take a walk in a park you've never visited, write a letter (on paper) and mail it to a friend, or better yet call up that friend and meet them at the new coffee shop.

If you spend all of your free time doggedly stewing over or researching ways to beat your current bugaboo—whether it be an illness, a problem at work, or a rift with a friend—set it aside for a few hours or even a few days.

Like any vacation, eventually we must return home, but if we take our mind on vacation for a time, we're often able to see our current home and its challenges with different eyes. So no matter where your vacation is, the most important item on your vacation packing list is you—body, mind, and soul.

Seeking a Second Opinion

August 10, 2012

~~~~~

I finally sought a second opinion on my Parkinson's diagnosis. After trying three different medications (which have not helped any of my symptoms and have caused side effects), the mind begins to wonder whether the diagnosis was correct, whether there are any other options, and whether you can really live with this new "normal" for the rest of your life.

I have gone back and forth on the issue of getting a second opinion. I didn't do it immediately because I just couldn't take one more doctor's appointment or test. The stress of insurance hassles and having to take half a day or more to spend time in a medical facility had no appeal to me. So, after doing my own research, I felt like I would trust my neurologist's diagnosis for the time being.

But one of the more terrible aspects of having a chronic, non-life-threatening condition is that you have lots of time to think and wonder about it—especially when you are a teacher and have the summer off from work. Enough doubts and concerns had niggled their way into my mind that I wanted someone who specialized in movement disorders to weigh in on the matter. The best option I found was a three-hour drive away.

When I called to make an appointment, I imagined it would take months to fit me in since I do not have a life-threatening illness. Not so. This particular hospital tries to get new patients an appointment within seven business days. I couldn't make it there for a same-day appointment, so they found a doctor who had an opening the next day.

I didn't have a lot of time to collect the necessary test results, but the local hospital pulled everything together for me within an hour or so of calling them. I tried to spend some time going over what I felt were the most important questions and issues that I wanted to discuss with the doctor because I didn't think I would have much time to talk to him, given my experiences in the past.

My two biggest fears were contradictory:

- He would say I did have Parkinson's disease.
- He would say I didn't have Parkinson's disease. It was something worse.

Of course, I also held onto the shred of hope that he would say, no, you don't have any terrible disease at all.

The appointment ended up being an all-day adventure since it involved six hours of driving round trip. All told, the neurologist and his staff spent more than one-and-a-half hours with me. I had plenty of time to ask questions. So what was the outcome?

The neurologist concurs with the original diagnosis that I have Parkinson's. Because there are no lab tests that can detect Parkinson's, doctors can only make a clinical diagnosis, so there is always that outside chance it is something else (like an atypical Parkinsonism). This neurologist thought it was unlikely in my case.

So what can I do? He gave me the following options:

- Because I am young and my symptoms are not interfering with my everyday activities, I don't need to take medication. I will have to live with the symptoms, but I won't end up with the nasty side effects of the medications.
- If the tremor becomes troublesome, there is a class of drugs that primarily targets the tremor. If I wanted something to take on an as-needed basis, say for an especially important presentation or event, I could look into trying one of them.

- He also knew of an observational clinical trial I might qualify for if interested.

He told me so much more, but that's enough for this venue. Even though I had heard or read much of the information before, the fact that he listened and gave me options was helpful. He didn't press me to make any decisions on the spot, but I did say that I was leaning toward the first option right now, as I prefer not taking unnecessary medications. I am still chewing on the idea of the clinical trials.

So was the drive, the time, and the cost worth getting a second opinion since it didn't effectively change anything?

In my case, yes. Doctors are intelligent and well-educated, but in the end they are people. When up against a disease as tricky and elusive as Parkinson's, doctors have much to offer the patient but still don't know everything or else there would be a cure. Allowing more than one person to weigh in on the diagnosis brings an entirely different set of experiences into the mix. While I hoped for a clean bill of health instead of confirmation of the disease, the niggling uncertainties are somewhat diminished.

Someday, I'll likely need medications or other interventions, but for now, I am going to see how far living life as healthily as I can will take me on this journey, while continuing to keep an ear out for alternative therapies and research breakthroughs.

Pity Party from 9–10

August 25, 2012

〜〜〜〜〜

Some may wonder if I have bad days since I try to keep the posts on my blog positive or at least neutral in attitude. So here's the longish answer to that question.

While I believe the worst (physically) is yet to come—short of a miraculous cure or healing—some days I want to say enough is enough and turn back the clock to a time when I had no complaints about the workings of my body. Surely, there is a magic bean or a time turner or wardrobe or something out there that can take me where I want to go and make my body be what I want it to be.

I have had some days like that recently. It is easy for me to clam up and not share about the more trying times because at some point in my childhood I internalized Thumper's mother's advice, "If you can't say something nice, don't say nothin' at all."

I am not sure how this happened, as I don't remember watching Bambi in its entirety. Somehow, I twisted this sentence from being a mother's attempt to teach self-control to mean that it is never okay to talk about the hard stuff of life.

Oops! I just said all those things. As I read back through them, I realize they aren't all that shocking or rude. They are realities for someone dealing with young-onset Parkinson's disease, and accepting that I am now living in the best days of the rest of my physical life is tough.

One way I know I am finally growing up is that difficult thoughts like these tend to be momentary rather than ongoing struggles. Though I have a melancholy temperament, I have learned not to dwell too long on the negatives life throws at me.

Many years ago, I received a bit of advice that boils down to, "Limit the length of your pity parties." We need to acknowledge the parts of our lives that expose our deepest fears and sadness and allow ourselves time to grieve our losses—including the loss of health. But it is not in our best interest to spend life as if we are attending a perpetual pity party. Parkinson's or not, I prefer not to be a resident of the State of Self Pity.

So, yes, I have bad times physically and emotionally. I worry, I get angry, I get exhausted, I cry, and on occasion, I pout. It's my pity party, and I'll cry if I want to because we can't have a stiff upper lip all the time. But I also have learn that if the invitation says "Party 9-10," I must do my best to end that pity party promptly at ten. Life consists of so much more than pity parties.[1]

---

[1] Disclaimer: No clichés were harmed in the writing of this post. The author believes in equal opportunity for most turns of phrase including clichés, puns, and applicable song titles.

THE SEASON OF DOING

September 12, 2012

~~~~~~

I don't have much time to post on the blog these days. The semester has begun, and I am teaching a full-time load for the first time in years. This seems a bit backwards when you think about it. I am diagnosed with a chronic, degenerative disease and then I decide to go back to work full time. Girl, what were you thinking?

Going back to work full time was something I thought I would do when my children were not home all day. (Because I homeschooled one or both of them up until two years ago, I put that change off longer than most.) Then my Parkinson's diagnosis called that plan into question, and I put all dreams on hold while I regrouped. In some ways, it felt as if my life was ending, and I discovered that when mortality comes and sits across the breakfast table from you, your appetite changes.

A Parkinson's diagnosis does not slide a poisoned cup of sudden death across the table to you. Instead, it slips a slow-acting poison into your breakfast each morning, shutting you down slowly and methodically, one brain cell at a time. All the while your uninvited guest sits across the table from you watching it happen with a sick smile on its face.

As those brain cells turn traitor, you despair that the rest of your life will be the equivalent of a never-ending succession of gruel, dry toast, and watery, lukewarm tea (or worse yet, coffee) with the buffet of life in eyesight but out of reach. I had my chance to partake of life, but

I didn't take advantage of the feast sitting before me the entire time.

While this may seem a bit over the top, these thoughts and feelings are simply a part of what I have experienced during this first year. When Parkinson's hits at a younger age, it forces you to gaze into a crystal ball and see your future with more clarity than most, yet giving in now because of what *may be* is not the answer.

And so I live. Not a day goes by that I forget I have been diagnosed with Parkinson's, but now that I have decided I can enter the "season of doing" despite my un-invited shadow, there are more and more moments and even hours when I can focus on the health I have. I am on the verge of letting my youngest fly on his own. Change is wisping into our lives, and my "season of doing" work outside of the home has arrived.

- I accepted a full-time teaching appointment for this year.
- I spent my summer trying to fulfill some of my more creative goals.
- I am considering other activities that will stretch me emotionally, spiritually, and physically.

Most surprisingly, I have found I can sometimes look across the table and smile at mortality—because it has reminded me I have a reason to live.

Pop Quiz Which Comes First: Stress or Parkinson's?

November 21, 2012

~~~~~~

A woman walks to the front of a group to make a report about an assignment she completed. She trembles violently as she begins to talk. The conclusion?

> A. *She must be nervous.*

A woman is waiting to play for a worship service. It is her first time playing with this particular band, and someone observes her shaking. Conclusion?

> A. *She must be nervous.*

It would be entirely reasonable for nerves to get the better of her in either situation, but how many multiple choice exams have you taken where there is only one answer? Probably not many. Yet, when it comes to making assumptions about the cause of a particular effect, we prefer to fill in the blank with the answer we think is most likely.

So what if both scenarios added a second option?

> A. *She must be nervous.*
> B. *She has young-onset Parkinson's disease.*

That changes things, but is the answer A or B? Since she always has a tremor because of the Parkinson's disease, the answer could be B.

Actually, as someone who has experienced both of these scenarios, I would like to add a third choice:

A. She must be nervous.
B. She has young-onset Parkinson's disease.
C. Both A and B

The cause of the tremor in both cases is a chicken-and-egg conundrum because stress can increase the symptoms of Parkinson's, but the tremor is persistent if not constant. I rarely shake as violently as I did when I gave the presentation, so I have to believe nervousness exacerbated the tremor. When I was waiting to play keyboard for the first time in a long time, I was excited but had practiced thoroughly. I did not feel nervous enough to tremble, so I concluded that my mild shakes were my usual Parkinson's tremor.

So which is the correct answer? Maybe we need a fourth option:

D. It depends on the situation.

THE FIRST ANNIVERSARY

November 30, 2012

~~~~~~

Today is an anniversary.

Though an anniversary usually invites celebration, I think you'll understand if I don't order a cake or bring out the champagne for this one Yet, I can't ignore this major turning point in my life.

It has been a year since a doctor first suspected I had Parkinson's disease. While it wasn't confirmed for another month or so, he was confident of his diagnosis that first day. Despite living with a diagnosis of Parkinson's, this year has been remarkably positive when it comes to the issue of health.

- My current symptoms are manageable, especially since I don't have the side effects of the medications to deal with.

- My left side still has a tremor and sometimes misbehaves or feels weak; however, the general fatigue and insomnia I have experienced at times seem to be less bothersome.

- I have been more conscientious about exercising regularly. I have logged 438 miles of running/walking since last Christmas, and I can easily jog two-and-a-half miles or more when my left foot cooperates and doesn't cramp up. I am trying to decide whether I can hit five hundred miles by Christmas or New Year's. We'll see. (If only I hadn't forgotten to take my iPod on some long hikes, I would be there!)

I list these facts not to brag but to remind myself to focus on the positives. It helps me to take out these reminders and hang them in the dark parts of my mind like a string of Christmas lights as a reminder that each year has its darkness, but it can be overcome if we plug in the lights.

LOWERING THE DOSE

December 6, 2012

~~~~~

Y ou'd expect this post to focus on medication, but that is not the case. I came to a realization a couple of months ago—I was overdosing on news about Parkinson's disease.

In the pre-Internet days, I was a library junkie. I sampled unaffordable subscriptions in the periodicals section, and then moved to the headier stuff found in the stacks. I could navigate a card catalog like a pro, but more often than not, I consulted the Dewey Decimal or Library of Congress Classifications, headed to a section of interest, and browsed. I always appreciated a library that had no check-out limitations, and when I wanted to know something, I lugged home a shelf of books for the prescribed loan period.

Then, the Internet happened. I kept up my library habits during its infancy, as the information on the Internet was always spotty and suspect, but now, I often go half a year or more between library visits with the event of more reliable sites and e-books.

As a part of my transition to Internet-based information sources (somewhere around the turn of the century), I discovered Google. One of Google's "still more" features is Google Alerts. You can plug in any search term, tell the search engine how often you want to hear about the topic, and Google magically delivers news on the subject to your e-mail inbox. When I began to research Parkinson's, I set up a daily Google Alert, but lately, it has gotten to be too much.

Many mornings, I would see a promising headline in the daily digest and eagerly read the article, only to find a rehash of old news or a breakthrough that had only been observed in mice. I could see myself becoming that woman from the pre-Internet era who missed life because she waited by the mailbox for the sweepstakes entries and mailed them back the next day because each one promised the possibility of winning the big one—someday. Living your life focused on what *may be* has drawbacks.

Rebel that I am, I lowered my dose of Parkinson's news without consulting a doctor. I didn't turn off my Google Alert completely, but I set it to once a week. I want to keep up with research advances but don't need to read about them every day.

As a result, I have lowered your dose, as well, because I don't post on my blog, *A Path Not Chosen*, as often as I did when I was bingeing on Parkinson's news.

My advice? Get out and enjoy life. When news of the big one—a true cure for Parkinson's—arrives, you won't need a Google alert to let you know. It is unlikely you will be able to miss the din of the millions of Parkinson's patients and their loved ones celebrating.

Exploring Alternative Routes

The Second Year

"I do not know," said the...[Wizard of Oz]; "but that is my answer, and until the Wicked Witch dies you will not see your uncle and aunt again. Remember that the Witch is Wicked—tremendously Wicked— and ought to be killed. Now go, and do not ask to see me again until you have done your task."
~L. Frank Baum, *The Wonderful Wizard of Oz*

By the end of 2012, I was determined to go without medications as long as I could, but I still felt like something needed to be done to deal with the enemy within me. I began to explore alternative ways people were trying to deal with Parkinson's.

After I had finished up the spring semester of classes, I chose not to return to teaching the next year, primarily because the commute was too long, but also to reduce my stress levels, which exacerbated my symptoms.

Early in 2015, I discovered a medical doctor who had a clinic that offered alternative therapies, and I made an appointment. He had me take a number of supplements to promote brain health and suggested chelation therapy, which is used to remove heavy metals from the body. In addition to the Parkinson's, I wanted to explore my ongoing allergies, and that process led to an elimination diet to see if I had any sensitivities to foods.

The result of my year of finding alternative ways to achieve my goals—to defeat my enemy and return home to the land of good health—were mixed. What follows are a few notes about the mental and emotional battles I faced in the second year living with Parkinson's.

UNWELCOME GUEST, MR. P.D. THE CAT

January 3, 2013

~~~~~

After I went for the second opinion in August 2012 and received the go ahead to stop taking all medications, I had a mental shift in the way I viewed Parkinson's. I can never escape the uncomfortable feeling I am like a mouse forced to give food and lodging to a cat with the dubious name, Mr. P.D. For the past few months, this uninvited boarder has been lying low, and I have done my best to ignore his presence. Next week, however, I have a follow-up exam with my original neurologist, and I can't ignore the old chap (Mr. P.D.) any more. To say I am dreading the visit is an understatement.

Because of the distance, the doctor (of the second opinion) suggested I keep my local neurologist. Since getting the second opinion and stopping my prescription, I haven't consulted with the original neurologist, and I feel a bit like a naughty child playing one parent against the other, even though I had every right to get the second opinion. Why the dread?

- I don't want to explain that I stopped taking the last prescription because someone else told me I didn't have to take it.
- I don't want to be told that things are not better or are worse.
- I don't want to fight against another prescription that I am sure he will recommend.

My visits to the doctor usually leave me wondering when I'll move from being the host at dinner to the roast for dinner. I hold out hope that some night Mr. P.D.

will slip out the door of my life as silently as he slipped in. Yet when I have reality checks like a doctor's appointment or an encounter with another Parkinson's patient who is further down the road than me, I remember that though Mr. P.D. is a patient killer, he can't help playing with his food. (But you can be very sure that I'll make Mr. P.D. Cat work hard for his dinner.)

THE STROOPWAFEL THAT BROKE THE MOUSE'S RESOLVE

January 26, 2013

Author's note: If you have never eaten a stroopwafel *(syrup waffle), a Dutch dessert, you must try one. Take a trip to your grocery store's international food aisle, order a package online, or book a vacation to the Netherlands for the most authentic treats. Once you've experienced a* stroopwafel *for yourself, you'll have a better understanding of the trauma a* stroopwafel *caused on an otherwise unremarkable day in January.*

Yes, it was an unremarkable day. I was working at home as classes had not yet started up for the semester, and my husband came home for lunch. We had some unremarkable leftovers, and then my husband disappeared into the pantry. Seconds later, I heard the crackle of the *stroopwafel* bag. He had been on a trip and managed to pick up a couple of packages as a treat. We don't usually have dessert with our lunch, but when *stroopwafels* are in the house, we make an exception.

If you did not take my advice and have never had the fortune of having a warm *stroopwafel* melt on your tongue, then I will try to fill you in, but reading about eating and eating are two distinctly different activities and one is far superior to the other. These Dutch desserts are best fresh, but the packaged ones will do. They consist of a thin waffle that is miraculously split in two and filled with a brown-sugar, caramel-like filling. The waffles are a little crisp on the outside, but the filling makes them slightly soft on the inside. While they are fine at room temperature, warming them slightly by perching them on top of a hot drink or placing them in the microwave for a few seconds almost duplicates eating them fresh.

I chose to warm mine in the microwave that fateful day. I was chatting with my husband and cleaning up from lunch while I awaited the goodness to come.

Moments (and yes, I mean *moments*) later, my husband asked if something was in the oven. Turning around, I saw black smoke pouring out of the microwave. I had automatically punched in two minutes, the length of time it takes to heat a cup of water in our microwave. The *stroopwafel* had only needed ten to fifteen seconds.

As I observed the blackened, smoking puck of previously-beautiful sugar and butter and all things lovely, I lost it. I had ruined a *stroopwafel* because I wasn't thinking. I was losing my memory! I couldn't focus! It was all because of the Parkinson's, and I was sick and tired of being sick and tired. Now a burned *stroopwafel* was causing me to have a nuclear meltdown.

But why? I have broken glasses and heirloom platters. I have ruined supper. I have burned the pancakes. While it would be easy to blame the *stroopwafel*, in the end it was just the innocent and proverbial straw that broke me like that ill-fated camel with the broken back.

The truth is, that unremarkable day was the day after my checkup with the doctor. The visit wasn't that bad. He didn't scold me (despite going behind his back for a second opinion). He didn't push me to go on medication, although he highly recommended that I do more research on one. I asked him point-blank if he thought my symptoms were worse than they were when he first diagnosed me, and he said they weren't. He said I didn't need another check-in for eight months. All good, right?

But here's the thing. Throughout the short examination, he kept repeating one statement, "This will progress."

Being reminded of that over and over again after trying to live life and ignore Mr. P.D. laid a heavy burden on this mouse's back. Should I be trying more medications? Should I more aggressively pursue some of the alternative therapies that are out there? What if I lose my ability to move? My ability to think?

While I have friends and family and even strangers giving me support, there are moments that a small reminder like, "It will progress," can make you feel so terribly alone even with a loved-one's arms wrapped tightly around you. It is a back-handed way of saying, "There's really nothing you can do."

The smoke's still clearing from that incident—at least within my soul. I am still struggling to know whether it is best to approach the future by accepting this as a cross to carry, a battle to be fought, or somewhere in between the two.

For now, you've heard the story of an otherwise unremarkable Wednesday when we happened to have *stroopwafels* in the house, and how they broke this mouse's resolve (at least for a time).

(And just so you know, the sacrificial *stroopwafel* was fortunately not the last—at least on that otherwise unremarkable day.)

Violet Days Will Come Again

May 1, 2013

~~~~~~

C olor. It is one of the things I like best about spring. Yesterday morning I opened the blinds and a sea of violets bathed in morning light greeted me. I couldn't resist heading out into the dew-drenched grass to do a photo shoot of my violet-dappled lawn. Violet days like these are rare. This showing won't survive the executioner's blade during the next much-needed mowing. But I am staying the execution at least one more day.

You can't have too many violet days.

I have had a few of my own violet days in the past couple of weeks—days where I pushed past winter's grayness and could hold my head up and honestly say, "I feel better than I have in a long time." Spring and sunlight have something to do with that. And so do the addition of some supplements, a change in diet, and more regular morning runs and exercise.

The article, "Not Just Tremor: Recognizing depression and other non-motor symptoms of Parkinson's disease,"[1] reminded me that truly good days for those with Parkinson's disease may be as few and fleeting as violet days in spring. For those who battle the darkness of depression and anxiety, or who withdraw from life, gray winter days can persist throughout the year. The grayness becomes the norm, and you begin to live as if it is a gray-scale world.

---

1 Valeo, Tom. "Not Just Tremor: Recognizing depression and other non-motor symptoms of Parkinson's disease." *Neurology Now.* Dec.-Jan. 2012 8(6), p 22–27.

Color does not seem to be an option, and you distrust those who try to tell you otherwise.

That is what makes violet days so special when they do crop up. They are reminders that even though our brain's color ink cartridges may be running low, it doesn't mean we've been transported to Dorothy's Kansas, a world devoid of hue. We don't have to travel to Oz to live in Technicolor. The color's still there, even when it is sometimes beyond our ability to see it.

So take a look out your back window and enjoy your violet days.

More Than a Shadow

May 17, 2013

~~~~~~

As I was walking through my dining room a few days ago, I saw that the sun had cast perfect silhouettes on the wall opposite a window that hosts a collection of herbs and bottles. Grey on beige, only the delicate outlines resembled the objects that cast the shadows.

Some days, we can feel like shadows of what we were before—*before* that big failure, *before* that failed relationship, *before* a chronic illness began to suck the color from our life.

Moments after I snapped a picture, the shadow on the wall had disappeared, but the objects on the window sill remained. Shadows are only unattached in Peter Pan. In reality, shadows depend on someone or something that *is*.

Maybe the light source has moved and our shadows have become darker or more pronounced, but no matter how it feels, if we see a shadow, a source exists. We are more than our shadow.

The Body I Thought I Knew

July 5, 2013

~~~~~~

E very so often, you're filling out a form and "they" want to know how you would rate your health on a 5-point scale from "1-Comatose on the couch" to "5-So excellent my body is the prototype for the superhero of the future."

When I have answered questions like these, I always think I am a 5, but I check "4-As good as it gets" because it seems presumptuous to claim that I am the epitome of health when I do break down and visit the doctor from time to time, hoping that I'll be the lucky patient who arrives on the day they finally reveal the cure to the common cold. In short, I have always thought of myself as a healthy person.

The events of the last decade have cast doubt on what I thought I knew about my body. My past mantra was, "If it looks and behaves as it should, everything under the hood must be in order." But with my Parkinson's diagnosis, I realized my body had been secretly organizing a coup for a number of years. I should have known something was going on right behind my eyes, but I didn't have a clue.

After the disheartening check-in with the neurologist in January, I felt like I couldn't do anything but wait for my life to get worse. That attitude was a major hope-sucker. In addition, I can't shake the feeling that somewhere, somehow, my body holds the answers to why I ended up with Parkinson's at a relatively young age.

So I finally decided to explore some alternative or complementary therapies people have tried in an effort to do something.

I found a medical doctor who is not far from where I live and is part of an association that incorporates alternative and complementary (as in additional—not free) therapies into their practice. This was a bit of a leap for me, but I decided all I had to lose initially was a morning's time and the fee to see the doctor.

That initial appointment was four weeks ago. As I had hoped, the doctor spent quite a bit of time looking at my health from a more holistic point of view, and after some discussion, my husband and I decided to go ahead and have several tests run.

I went back to discuss the results of those tests, and I have now been given several things to do. It seems I was right not to check a five on those general health questions. The results show that I have several underlying issues that may or may not contribute to my Parkinson's and chronic allergies, but over the next few months, we will see if addressing them makes a difference in my overall health.

The first three items on my list:

- Try to pinpoint potential food sensitivities/allergies through an elimination diet. [For now, goodbye to wheat/gluten, dairy, eggs, yeast, and (of all things) pineapple.]
- Start taking vitamin supplements.
- Go through chelation therapy, a process to reduce the toxic metals in my system.

That's enough to keep me busy for the next couple of months. We'll see if there are any noticeable changes or if I have committed myself to a Sisyphean task in pursuit of the body I thought I had and would like returned to me.

Do you really want to get well?

August 7, 2013

~~~~~~

Let's start with a confession. (I am sure this doesn't apply to you and yours, but indulge me.)[1]

Sometimes when the pastor is reading scripture during a worship service my mind wanders. The more familiar the passage is, the longer the journey. I have been there, done that, and have the T-shirt. (Or at least some member of the youth group does.)

Believe me, I am not proud of this, but it is the truth.

When my mind is tempted to meander, one way I try to refocus is to read between the lines or to pick up a familiar word or phrase and look at it from a different angle. (Have no fear, I am not trying to add anything to scripture, but both you and I know that even in Bible times, people probably talked a lot more and did a lot more than scripture lets on. I am also certain that they did not insert chapter and verse numbers into their everyday conversations, as Bible publishers seem to indicate, but I digress.) Another technique I sometimes use is to put myself in the place of one of the characters.

Several months ago, the familiar story of the man healed by the pool of Bethesda (John 5:1-15) was the scripture of the day at my church. You may know it. It goes something like this (in Sherri's paraphrased version):

> *A man would lie by a pool with healing waters every day. He'd been lame for thirty-eight years. Every so often, the waters of the pool stirred. He*

---

1 Originally published on the Churches of God Women's Ministries Blog, *WomenforGod.org*. 7 Aug. 2013

> *could have been healed if he had gotten into the*
> *pool first, but no one would help him. One day*
> *Jesus came by and healed him. The man got up*
> *and walked, (and the Jewish leaders celebrated*
> *by scolding him for getting healed and carrying*
> *his mat on the Sabbath).*

This story, and what follows it, focuses on Jesus' miracle and his ongoing conflict with the Jewish leaders. The miracle, minus the conflict, is the story I learned so many years ago in Sunday School with vintage presentation software—the flannelgraph. That Sunday morning in February, my mind was in danger of wandering off when I heard the familiar story, but then I noticed how much was left unsaid. And for the first time, I could identify with the lame man, as I had just passed the first anniversary of my diagnosis of Parkinson's disease.

I imagined myself lying on that mat for thirty-eight years of my life among so many others who also wanted healing but were more mobile or had more friends than I did.

That group of misfits would become like family because I wasn't the only one who had missed the chance to be healed over and over again, and yet they were also my competitors. Rivalry and bitterness crept in. At some point, the humiliation of my disability had given way to resignation of its norm, but that didn't keep me from complaining about my lot in life to anyone who would listen.

One day a teacher with a northern accent came along, picked me out of the crowd and asked, "Do you want to get well?"

I couldn't believe the nerve of the guy. Who doesn't want to be well? And why else would I be hanging out at this pool if I didn't want healed?

After a moment of staring at him, a faint hope flitted inside. He seemed compassionate and strong. Maybe he would sit down and wait with me until the next opportunity for healing. But a familiar uneasiness at the unknown world of health brushed that aside, and familiar complaints whined out of my lips. "I am too slow to get into the water when it moves, and no one will help me."

I expected to hear the clink of a coin on stone or a look of disgust or pity. Instead, he said something that I had only ever heard as a cruel joke, "Get up and walk."

Then the story simply says the man was healed, gathered up his mat, and walked away. I found that I couldn't imagine what he was thinking following this surprising command. We usually assume a person would leap up in joy like the lame man healed by Peter and John in Acts 3, but there is no mention of a thank you. And apparently the man didn't even ask Jesus what his name was before Jesus slipped away. He only finds out later after being slapped on the hand by the Jewish leaders for carrying his sleeping mat on the Sabbath. Jesus later warns him to stop sinning, and the man repays Jesus by revealing his identity to his enemies.

So we're left to read between the lines in the last part of the story. Did the man suddenly realize that healing wouldn't fix everything and that he was more comfortable being the lame man who couldn't get a break? Were praise and gratitude like foreign languages and too difficult to learn at his age? Was a healthy future too frightening? Had he indulged in deception or self-pity for so long that he did not know how to quit?

We really don't know the rest of the lame man's story. But we do know ours. Some of us live with chronic or terminal illnesses. Others have healthy bodies. But when it comes down to it, we are all in need of spiritual healing, and the question we have to ask ourselves is the same one Jesus asked the lame man: Do we really want to get well?

Be Kind to Silly Putty

October 3, 2013

~~~~~~

I woke up on the verge of crying this morning. Don't ask me why or what I dreamed about because I don't remember. A predawn run and its accompanying endorphin squad soon brought the potential flood under control. The upshot of the odd start to the day?

I realized we should be kinder to Silly Putty.

Yes, the mind works in mysterious and incredibly strange ways. Is it more bizarre to wake up crying or to suddenly develop a compassion for a non-sentient, viscous substance that compels us to play with it, mold it, stretch it, bounce it, break it, and press newspaper ink onto it?

That is a question. (Whether or not it deserves an answer is another non-grammatical subject altogether.)

Why this sudden campaign to end Silly Putty abuse?

Even though I don't know the precise reason I woke up in the middle of an emotional rain cloud, when I find myself in one, the heart is usually involved, and I don't mean "a blood-pumping organ in an animate being." I mean the seat of our emotions—that intangible ticker that keeps us putting one foot in front of the other each day, even though some days we feel it has been played with, re-molded, stretched thin, bounced silly, broken into a million pieces, and impressed with the ink of so many relationships it is now a gray ball we no longer recognize.

Hearts and Silly Putty—they are both resilient, but they go through a lot, don't they?

That's why I think we should be kinder to Silly Putty.

STEPPING BACK FROM WORRY
October 29, 2013

~~~~~~

Last week, I was reading a health forum discussing whether or not to discontinue a medication. I was surprised to see the thread had become one contributor's personal medical log as he weaned himself off that medication (with his doctor's oversight). While I could see the benefit of his meticulous detail, as some medications are quite difficult to fine-tune, I felt stressed by the time I had flipped through the pages and pages of posts because I don't know if I could ever focus on a health issue in such detail—even if my life depended on it.

In the interest of full disclosure, I can be a detail-oriented person who will hunt down the one penny keeping my checkbook from balancing, but even I have limits despite being a recovering perfectionist. When it comes to health, I can log and chart and keep track of symptoms for a while, but after a time the process is not only tedious but counter-productive. The constant attention I give to the disease or health issue leads to one of the foundations of worry—focusing too much on temporal, physical needs—which I have come to think of as the "dots" in our life's pointillist painting.

We need those dots to be sure. If you believe that all we have is the present and life ends when our body gives out, it makes sense to do what you can to prolong the journey by paying attention to the details. But whether or not life extends beyond this reality (which I believe it does), what kind of trip will it be if we spend our days worrying about the dots of life as if we are trying to get the best fuel economy out of our vehicle 24-7? Are the tires inflated just so? Should I drive 56.7 miles per hour or 67.4 miles per hour? Would a fuel additive help or can I convert my engine so that it runs on garbage like a *Back-to-the-Future* DeLorean? If we never step back from the "dots," we can begin to think our body's physical needs are all there is to life.

Though I am thankful to each person who has made a difference in the world by paying attention to the details of life, I start to get cross and a bit cross-eyed if I stare at the dots too closely for too long. Worry begins when I focus only on details and don't take a step back from time to time, allowing myself to see how the dots connect to create meaning, perspective, color, and beauty—what life should be.

A Flash of Fall Fire

November 4, 2013

~~~~~~

I thought the colors of fall would not come to my corner of the world this year. I expect them in early to mid-October, but many trees humbly lost their leaves without any hue-full fanfare. And others donned only muted mustards and browns. So a couple of weeks ago, I swallowed my disappointment and hoped for a better show next year. But it seems I was too impatient as fall is fashionably late and a bit shy with patches of scarlet and orange turning up here and there during this first week of November.

Yesterday morning, I arose before sunrise thanks to the return to Standard Time. As I was reading the morning news in my second-story perch, I thought I saw a flame outside. I looked up to see the tree tops on fire with fall color.

I am glad I captured the instant in a photo. Though it does not do justice to what I saw, it hints at it, and the color did not last. Moments later, the morning sun continued to rise, and the trees returned to their duller yellows, greens, and browns.

The light made all of the difference.

In the Beginning There Were No Doctors

November 14, 2013

~~~~~~

Are my expectations of doctors fair? That is the question that I find myself gnawing on after a less-than-fulfilling check in with the neurologist yesterday morning.

As I stepped out of the doctor's office into the November chill (an hour and a half later than I had planned), I was already working on a blog post in my mind. It starred me as the victim of a health system gone wrong and featured a riveting plot designed to let you feel my pain and exasperation second by second. (And I would have had to fill you in on each second to have a full-length post as the exam only lasted around five to ten minutes.)

It was good that I needed to pick up groceries before heading home because it allowed me to chill long enough to remember this:

In the beginning, there were no doctors.

Sit back and think about that for just a moment. Whether you think humans sprung from the creative Word of God or slithered out of the primordial ooze, none of the stories of man's earliest days mention an award-winning hospital complete with ICU and trauma care, much less an obstetrician to deliver the babies. They couldn't dial 911 and have a crew of paramedics come to their rescue. They didn't have government-funded research facilities trying to find cures for every disease known and unknown to man. They didn't even have the most rudimentary of doctor's offices on the corner. If a person was ill or injured, they did what little they knew to do, but ultimately had to leave their health and life in the hands of God or fate or whatever higher power they believed in.

This perspective check made me think that maybe, just maybe, the expectations I had for my check up were a bit myopic and idealistic.

- Perhaps, after researching and stewing over and living with my "issues" for months, it is unreasonable to expect a doctor to have much sympathy when he's seen so many patients during that time that he can't remember who I am until he reviews my chart.
- Perhaps, when there are so many people waiting at his door to see him, it is selfish to think that I need more attention than any of them.
- Perhaps, it is illogical to keep going to a doctor expecting him to consider a radically different therapeutic approach than he has in the past.

And undoubtedly, it was wrong of me to sit in the examination room expecting God to walk in and shake my hand when I know the physician is simply a man.

I needed to be reminded that in the beginning, *there were no doctors.*

And the Word of the Year Is...

November 30, 2013

~~~~~~~~~~

Two years. That's how long it has been since I walked out of a neurologist's office with a probable diagnosis of Parkinson's disease. The first year was a time of learning, adjusting, and experimenting as I mentioned in last year's anniversary update.

While this year's challenges have continued to include experimentation with diet and detoxifying, I didn't gorge on research as much as I did the first few months after the diagnosis. I also realized recently that I have adjusted to my current symptoms in odd little ways. For example, if you see me crossing my arms, it rarely means I am angry, defensive, or insecure, as most people proficient in body language would suppose. This pose most likely has a less sinister meaning that has nothing to do with you. My hyperactive left arm often needs a time out under the firm protection of my still steady right arm. Crossing my arms when standing gives me some control over my most annoying symptom—the tremor.

If I had to sum up this past year's challenges in a word, I would pick *persevering*. Some days, *endure* would be the better word, as I haven't always wanted to keep going when I look down the road at my possible future. To endure implies that you have no choice in a situation and you just have to grin and bear it—or sob and curse it, depending on your preferred response.

But perseverance is different. *Dictionary.com* describes it as the ability to "maintain a purpose in spite of difficulty, obstacles, or discouragement." To me, that definition implies that even in the midst of circumstances I cannot control, I have choices. My life has not lost its meaning at the hands of a physical disease.

On the days when depression fogs my brain or an obstacle mires me in a pit of despair, I often lose sight of purpose and feel like I am simply enduring the moments that have been given to me. But thankfully, I have had enough violet days in 2013 to clear the view and remind me that purpose and meaning in life exists, allowing me to learn perseverance—even if the only purpose I can grasp is the dim memory that life is so much more than the dust of atoms and molecules that sometimes do not behave.

So in the spirit of persevering, here's to the next twelve months and whatever theme word they bring.

Do I Have To Keep Walking?

The Third Year

"If we walk far enough," said Dorothy, "I am sure we shall sometime come to some place." But day by day passed away, and they still saw nothing before them but the scarlet fields....Then Dorothy lost heart. She sat down on the grass and looked at her companions, and they sat down and looked at her, and Toto found that for the first time in his life he was too tired to chase a butterfly that flew past his head. So he put out his tongue and panted and looked at Dorothy as if to ask what they should do next.
~L. Frank Baum, *The Wonderful Wizard of Oz*

After a year of attacking my condition with alternative therapies, I had a follow-up appointment with my neurologist. That visit was as disappointing as Dorothy's second visit to the Wizard of Oz.

Even though she had killed the Wicked Witch as required, "Oz, the Great and Terrible" was revealed to be a balloonist from Omaha. When the Wizard managed to construct a balloon to help Dorothy escape the Land of Oz, it took off prematurely, and Dorothy found herself in search of a way home once again. A soldier in the Emerald City suggested she go see Glinda, the Witch of the South, who was a good witch. He thought she might be able to help Dorothy, but warned her that many dangers lay along the path to Glinda's lands.

Similarly, I still wanted to get home to my pre-Parkinson's existence, but nothing I tried helped. Some of my symptoms were getting worse.

In many of the books I read, the authors suggested working with a neurologist who specialized in Parkinson's or movement disorders. I had discovered a Parkinson's center less than an hour's drive from home, but I had two hesitations about going there. The first was the discomfort of asking for a referral from my neurologist. I also wondered if changing doctors would really make a difference since no cure exists. Yet this Parkinson's center was a part of a teaching hospital that was involved in research and clinical trials. If any breakthroughs happened, perhaps, I would learn about them sooner if I became a patient there.

I had come to a crossroads where I again had to make a choice not knowing whether any path could take me closer to my goal.

Which Way Should I Go?

February 2, 2014

~~~~~~

As I move into my third year of living with Parkinson's disease, I am standing at a crossroads again. If you happened to catch my rather cynical post, "In the Beginning There Were No Doctors," back in November, you'll know that I had an unsatisfying doctor's visit that day. And if you read my anniversary update on November 30, "And the Word of the Year Is...," I hinted at the internal conflict that visit stirred up, but I didn't go into detail.

That appointment once again stirred up the issue of whether I should be taking medication to alleviate my tremor and muscle rigidity. I am willing to live with my symptoms on most days, but some moments I wish I could escape into the healthy body I used to have. So once again, I am considering which path is the right one for me.

Option 1: Continue with Alternative Therapies

I spent 2012 trying alternative therapies. I finished a round of chelation therapy last summer and was able to reduce some of the heavy metals in my system. Some of the supplements I took were designed to help with detoxification and brain health. While they helped my overall health, they did not eliminate or reduce any of my Parkinson's symptoms. I had quite a collection of supplements by fall, and I didn't know what was doing what. As they have run out, I have not renewed my supply. My perception is that my symptoms may be slightly worse right now, but again, I am uncertain.

The main problem with continuing on this path is the cost. Many of the expenses for supplements and the various tests are out of pocket and not covered by insurance or medical reimbursement accounts. The doctor I have seen is not in our insurance network so, again, the cost could become more than our budget could bear, but I really want a doctor involved who is willing to think outside the box and pursue unconventional options.

Unreasonable cost also applies to other therapies I have read about like a space-age looking suit created by the Swedish company, Inervention, which is designed to help people with neurological problems, including Parkinson's Disease. Another potentially costly and frightening possibility is deep brain stimulation (DBS), which was something else mentioned in that last doctor's visit. I feel that it is too soon for a procedure that seems so risky, even though it has proved effective. Though DBS is becoming a standard therapy for Parkinson's Disease, I am not ready for that option.

Option 2: Re-Try Traditional Medications

One thing that people have said in response to hearing about my diagnosis is, "That's terrible, but they can do so much with medications these days." At the time, it gave me hope that with medications I could maintain a semblance of normal life for years or even a couple of decades. I spent the first eight months unsuccessfully trying three different medications that fall into two of the classes of drugs used to treat Parkinson's.

The drugs' side effects of sleeplessness, feeling like I was on a constant adrenaline rush, and having to watch what I ate (with one medication) weren't worth it when I couldn't move up to high enough doses to reduce my tremor or muscle rigidity in my left side.

Even though I have made it clear to my original neurologist that I don't want to go on medication, when I had a follow-up appointment, I wasn't allowed to leave the office without a prescription and a month's worth of samples. The medication is very expensive, even with a prescription plan, so I stuck the boxes in a cabinet and forgot about them for the most part.

I have to admit that I have had three days in the past couple of months when I was fed up enough by my tremor or the inability to relax my left arm and leg that I broke into the samples and tried the medication, which is administered through a patch worn 24 hours a day.

I haven't been able to leave one on for more than 12 hours. The first time, I developed a rash and nausea, and the last two times, I have woken up in the middle of the night with severe nausea, which resulted in vomiting. Needless to say, I am not inclined to try again, and though I haven't tried every possible medication, I am beginning to wonder if medications are going to be a viable option for me when I get to that stage when I may need them to function.

Option 3: Stay at the Crossroads for Now

A part of me just wants to focus on living a healthy lifestyle by continuing to exercise and exploring nutritional therapies, but after several months of eating a more restricted diet, I am not convinced that it directly affects the Parkinson's. I am losing my ability to play piano with my left hand, and typing can be a challenge. It is becoming more evident to me that staying at the crossroads and doing nothing may limit my ability to do the things I would like to do sooner rather than later.

Not So Very Brave

February 26, 2014

~~~~~

When I was in my early twenties, I met a woman who had recently been diagnosed with a chronic disease. I could summon up sympathy for her, but having never walked a similar path, I did not know what to do or say. From my very outside perspective, she appeared brave, and I told her so.

She said she was not so very brave.

I did not know how to respond at the time, but now I understand why she felt this way.

Courage is a choice. When you're on a path you did not choose, you are forced to face giants that you would have run from in another life. Just because you are shoved into the confrontation does not mean you are courageous. You can still cover your head and try to hide, even if you cannot run away. You can lie down on the path and allow the giant to do its worst. You can pout and cry, "It is not fair!" None of these choices is particularly courageous.

Not-so-brave days happen—sometimes turning into not-so-brave weeks or months. Sometimes all of the courage you can summon is to try to fall face up.

That Day Is Not Today: A Psalm of Complaint

Another day.

Some moments I believe I can still do
    whatever I want.
I am not going to let this disease stop
    me.
The next moment, I feel weak, useless,
    and finished.
How can I have a meaningful existence
    locked inside a body that won't be-
    have?

An unresponsive body gives me no
    choice.
Even if I find the courage to act,
I may not be able to do so.

But that day is not today.
It is a "what if" that may be circumvented
    by
A cure,
An effective therapy,
Or the end of life due to some other ail-
    ment or accident.

Each day.
It becomes harder and harder for me to
    lift myself out of this dark cup
To peer over its edge like Kilroy,
So that I can see beyond its sheer, slick
    sides
To the riot of life and love beyond it.

I am caught in a two-dimensional flat-
land
Where everything consists of lines of
various lengths.
The depth and breadth of life has vanished,
And it becomes harder to imagine other
planes exist.

This perception is cheered on by the un-
named evil that is killing off the cells in
my brain—
Starving me of dopamine,
The neurotransmitter of rewards.
This twisted enemy turns my own body
against me;
If it can keep me still and in the dark-
ness,
I will hasten my own demise.

What is the point of fighting
If there is no prize at the bottom of the
cereal box?

Today.
Even as I slip into the depths once again
With darkness on all sides,
A faint memory urges me to fall—looking
up.
I fold my eyelids into their place—some-
thing I can still do—
And see above me not a line but an oval.
An eye to another dimension, deep and
dotted with light.

Why Can't We Take Every Exit?

March 18, 2014

~~~~~~

The summer I was five, my father and I drove from Oklahoma to West Virginia together. On that long trip, I did not have digital entertainment, so I looked out the window to see what I could see. Howard Johnson's orange roofs and McDonald's golden arches caught my attention, and I remember asking him why we didn't get off at every exit because surely we were missing a lot by driving on by. He chuckled and told me that we would never get where we were going if we stopped at every exit.

Now that I am further down life's road and I take a moment to look back at where I have come from, I see the many exits that I never explored. Sometimes I question whether I should have slowed down and taken more time to investigate some of those paths. Like my five-year-old self, I wonder what treasures I failed to hunt down in my haste to arrive at my destination. And yet, if I had tried to explore every exit I passed, my father's simple, yet sage observation would have come true—I would not have gotten far.

As it often does, the answer lies somewhere in between the vagabond who meanders aimlessly and the anti-traveler whose only goal is to get from Point A to Point B in the shortest time possible. No, we can't stop at every exit, but when we do pull off the highway and rest a while, we should take time for more than a sixty-second pit stop. You never know what treasures you might find along the way.

WHEN IT IS NOT OUR TIME
March 27, 2014

~~~~~~~~

A time for everything. Yet when mournful, depressing, or saddening times come, even for someone we only know through a Google news feed, it can sometimes seem that no other time can exist.

Should exist.

Will ever exist again.

When we are chastened by someone else's trials, and realize that by comparison our life is privileged, we bow our head and our heart—not always in humbleness but often with shame. It seems macabre and disrespectful to smile or enjoy or go on with our small lives. We do not sit in sack cloth and ashes—the dress of mourning—but on the stool in the corner in the most disturbing clown outfit we can imagine. Our cheeks are red, but not made up. How long is the time out? Five minutes? The duration that it takes to browbeat ourselves so we feel the others' pain? Until that moment when we believe we should not or cannot go on trying (and failing) to empathize any longer?

Yet, go on is what we must do. Each morning that breath re-enters our lungs, we must rise and take on the endeavor that awaits us. Some days the work is dull or the tasks are small. On others, joy froths out of the menial and laughter skips easily from our lips. Days will come when we must abandon one occupation for another. But many days, we grind along in the tracks we've worn through habit and duty because we don't know what else to do. Some call this tedium, others contentment and a place to belong.

I have often wondered what would happen if everyone in the world did something at the same time. For example, what if we all jumped and landed at the same time? Would the world wobble or be thrown off course? Would the force of our landing be canceled out by those that are opposite us?

It is an interesting thought experiment, but unlikely to happen. It is just not natural to be that synchronized. When we're told there is a time for everything, it does not mean that we will all be in lock-step doing and feeling and experiencing the same things at the same time. Life consists of melodies and counter melodies—syncopation and fugue. Our times do not always coincide, and I think that is a good thing.

We should laugh with those with reason to laugh and mourn with those we know are mourning, but we must hope ever so fervently that few events transpire where we all experience the same degree of loss or tragedy at the same moment. That way instead of hiding in the corner, ashamed that our life is not hard enough to truly empathize with our neighbor, we can simply know that is not our part to play at this particular moment. And when we are not one of the ones falling to the earth, perhaps, we can be there to break the fall or comfort those who are.

Why Should I Be Aware of All These Diseases?

April 1, 2014

~~~~~

If you're like me, you've asked the question, "Why should I be aware of all of the diseases that have awareness months?" Or maybe the sheer numbers overwhelm you, and the question is, "How can I be aware of all of these diseases?" You see the ribbons, the posters, the 5Ks, T-shirts, Facebook profile images, and so on and wonder how in the world these help fight a life-changing, life-threatening disease. Wouldn't it be better to funnel all of the funds and resources into actual research or medical care?

I am still asking these questions, but my attitude is changing since Parkinson's became a part of my life. Though I have yet to participate in any awareness events beyond starting this blog and writing about my journey, I think that all of the people who decide to raise awareness of a particular disease or disability have one thing in common—that challenge has touched them or someone that they know in some way.

It is not possible to be fully aware of every health challenge, but if you find yourself or someone you know engaged in a battle against a disease, here are some reasons why it is worth taking the time to learn more about the enemy.

KNOWLEDGE DESTROYS PREJUDICES AND MISUNDERSTANDINGS

You don't need to understand a disease at the molecular level, but understanding its symptoms and how it affects a person in daily life can help you break down your own prejudices and prevent misunderstandings. I have written about some of the ways people could misconstrue my body language now that I am trying to keep a tremor under control, and I am not alone in this. You may remember a story during the 2012 London Olympics where motor control issues common in Parkinson's were a factor in the arrest of a spectator. Awareness cannot prevent all occurrences of discrimination, but it has the potential to reduce them.

AN OUNCE OF AWARENESS COULD BE WORTH A POUND OF CURE (OR MORE)

Even though we cannot indefinitely prevent all diseases, it is in our nature to want to prolong life and be healthy. As researchers make new discoveries about the causes of common maladies, they often offer advice on how to prevent the problem in the first place. Keeping abreast of what is happening on the research front and making lifestyle choices that promote healthy living may help you avoid contracting certain diseases.

EVERY PLAYER NEEDS FANS

Seeing a disease as an opponent brings out our fight response, much as sporting events do. Like a football game, not everyone who is interested in defeating the opponent can be on the field, so they end up working behind the scenes in the locker room or writing a blog about their favorite team or watching in the stands or via television as fans.

Even though the role of fans can seem insignificant, without them the game changes. Sometimes it is the cheering of the masses or even just one key supporter that can keep a player from running off the field at a critical moment. I know this is true. If it weren't for my family, friends, and readers, some days I would not find the energy or courage to try one more way to slow down or reverse the enemy that is fighting against me on a daily basis. So thank you for becoming more aware of Parkinson's and supporting me.

When the World Seems Small
April 4, 2014

~~~~~~

The clouds press down this morning, shrinking the size of my world to a shell not much larger than my being. I cannot see beyond the twisting in my gut or the swelling of my tongue. Questions have been deployed to seek out the perpetrators of these world-diminishing attacks on my being—body and soul. Is it my arch-enemy or just an opportunistic sub-villain? No answers yet; all scouts have vanished into the fog.

So I wait.

The needs of my frail vessel expand like a bloated balloon to fill today's small world, but I don't think this is what Disney meant. After all, no matter how many people you stuff on a globe, they still cannot feel your pain, just as you cannot ever truly feel theirs. This corporeal tent only fits one.

Another peg loses its hold; I fight against the now misshapen canvas, pushing it back into place only for it to collapse once again. My lungs grasp for air in this claustrophobic environment, and I wish for those days when the world loomed large, wide, and flourishing with possibility—when I was not aware of the fragile crust that surrounds me.

I flip through the card file of cures that have disappointed, including the ace—faith in the God who shaped this craft that now has irreparable leaks. So far I've not been given any miraculous chewing gum to patch the holes in my health.

Despite my inability to see past the opaque shroud of my small world this morning, an infinitesimal tear sheds light, and I realize that we almost always question pain and rarely ask, "Why do good things happen?"

Old Fashioned vs. Instant Oatmeal Hope

April 4, 2014

"Parkinson's could soon be history post groundbreaking discovery"[1]

When I see this headline in my news feed a shot of hope thrills through me. I jab my mouse pointer on the promise-filled words, only to be disappointed again when I read that the breakthrough has occurred in fruit flies. I do a quick search for the original study or press release and skim through the contents on the John Hopkins website to find this:

"There's a big chasm between animal disease models and human treatments," says Ian Martin, Ph.D., a neuroscientist in Dawson's lab and the lead author on the paper. "But it is exciting. I think it definitely could turn into something real, hopefully in my lifetime."[2]

I don't know how old Dr. Martin is, but even if the research team discovers a treatment within the next five years, it would be optimistic to think that it could progress through animal and human trials in fewer than 10-15 years from the little I have observed of the research-to-treatment process. While I may live with Parkinson's longer than that, unless they find a treatment that can reverse the damage rather than simply stop the brain

---

1 "Parkinson's disease could soon be history post groundbreaking discovery," Science. *Business Standard.* Apr 11, 2014.
2 "Getting to the Root of Parkinson's Disease," *News and Publications.* Johns Hopkins Medicine. Apr 10, 2014.

from degenerating further, I will have 10-15 more years of damage to contend with if this treatment happens.

Don't get me wrong; what these scientists are doing and discovering is amazing and hopeful. I am glad I am dealing with this now and not one hundred years ago. But what their research offers is not an instant-oatmeal brand of hope—just add water and heal your disease.

That's what we all want, isn't it? And that's the brand of disappointing hope we end up with if we simply read the headlines and don't drill down to the body of truth behind them.

We can't be experts about everything and can only take in so much information each day, but one thing I have learned in trying to understand a chronic disease is that I have to avoid instant-oatmeal hope. Instead, I need an old-fashioned-oatmeal kind of hope. It is a slow-cooking, simmering hope that is willing to endure without giving in, despite the unknown cooking time required by some difficulties. It is a hope that doesn't pin the future to one outcome, but calmly delights in unknown potentialities and the belief that good ultimately triumphs over the not-good despite outward appearances.

So next time you see a promising headline, read on to find out what kind of hope lies behind it. And if you don't have time to do the research, avoid the urge to pass instant-oatmeal packets of hope on to those who are dealing with difficulty. Instead ask questions. Did you hear about this new treatment? What do you know about that study? Your friend may already know the answer or may decide to find out more. By asking questions, you show you're interested without offering false hope, and that can go a long way toward fostering the kind of old-fashioned oatmeal hope we all need.

The Stories We Tell Ourselves
April 25, 2014

Telling stories. Context changes the meaning of this phrase, doesn't it? Are we referring to a cozy bedtime activity or a lie? The ability of this one phrase to refer to actions that have widely different motivations and results reveals something of the power of story in our lives.

Stories can entertain, thrill, or frighten us. They can build someone up or tear another down. Stories undergird and inform our lives. *The stories we tell ourselves matter because the best stories reveal truth, but the worst perpetuate lies.* They affect the way we remember the past and look toward the future.

Take this story I told myself back in August 2013:

> *This weekend sucked. My husband was traveling, and my son and I, the two quietest and introverted members of our small family, whispered around the house like shadows.*

> *My body gave out on me physically and mentally. I woke up late on Saturday with no energy to do a morning run. I didn't have music for a new song I needed to learn for Sunday, so I spent two-and-a-half hours on Saturday morning working out the piano part by ear and running through the rest of the worship set. It was disheartening. My*

left hand really holds me back when I play piano thanks to Parkinson's.

Then, I was too tired to do anything but play an online game most of the afternoon. Sunday morning, the alarm woke me at six, and again, I determined I didn't have enough time or energy to exercise. By the time my son and I left for practice at eight a.m., I knew that my brain wasn't cooperating. My tremors were worse than usual, and I could not control the tension in my left side's muscles. A vicious circle began, and I couldn't escape. The situation caused stress, which caused my body to act up, causing me more stress.

I couldn't win, and I spent the rest of the morning just trying to make it through the practice and service without flooding tears all over the stage. I felt like such a hypocrite singing most of the songs. The pent-up emotions kept bursting out all afternoon. I knew I needed people, but no one needed me that day. And I was not fit company for anyone.

So again, I played an inane game that blanked out most of the rest of the day with only a few short interludes to get something to eat, take care of bodily necessities, and to help my son with a small problem. I managed to game away the entire day and went to bed at 9:45, falling asleep an hour or so

*later. A stupid waste of time, resources, and
time. I hate it when I do this.*

This story paints that weekend as torturous and life-sapping. And this is the story I told myself the following Monday morning. After writing the story down in my journal, I realized I hated the story. It needed a rewrite with a different point of view. I didn't like where the story was heading, and I didn't like the main character much.

Here's the re-telling:

> *This weekend was a challenge. My husband
> was traveling, but my son and I had time
> for rejuvenation after a week filled with in-
> teraction. We ate meals together, but other
> than that gave each other space to recharge
> our introverted batteries.*

> *I gave myself the weekend off from exercise
> and focused on getting more sleep. I had the
> opportunity to play for worship on Sunday,
> so I spent two-and-a-half hours on Satur-
> day morning figuring out a new song and
> running through the songs I already knew.*

> *I had thought I would tackle some writing
> projects over the weekend, but instead, I
> cashed in some stay-cation time and in-
> dulged in computer game playing—some-
> thing I rarely do.*

> *My son helped me make supper Saturday
> night, which we enjoyed together, and then
> on Sunday, I managed to rise at six, ready
> to leave for set-up and practice by eight*

without rushing. The practice went well. The band was ready to go right on time, and most of the songs only required one run through.

Despite my tremor acting up, I managed to get through the practice and worship times without any major catastrophes, and though I wish my stress levels had been lower so I could have enjoyed the experience more fully, I was able to cope and do what I needed to do.

After lunch out with my son, we retired to more relaxation. I tried out a new game that kept me interested until it was time for bed. I don't want to have many of these weekends, but it was time to recharge.

Though this rewrite may seem like a Pollyanna version that lacks the raw truthfulness of the first, are our negative feelings really the lowest common denominator in our experiences? Should we cast every experience in a pessimistic light because it seems more honest?

For those with a melancholy personality or who live with depression, the answer seems to be a resounding "yes." That is how we experience the world much of the time, and we don't trust those who tell stories that paint a picture of a sunny world. We tend to think optimists don't understand reality and delude themselves with their positive words.

Having lived in the shadows much of my life, I distrust full-scale, Technicolor optimism, but I have had enough glimpses of a world bathed in natural sunlight to know this is not a grayscale world. I realize the darkness can also lie to me. Even if the feelings I have are real, they often are brought on by falsehoods.

More and more, I am drawn to the color of truth, and the words I choose in the stories I tell myself either take me deeper into the shadows or edge me out into the light. The stories we tell ourselves matter.

THE NOT KNOWING

May 8, 2014

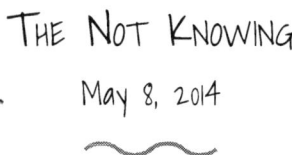

or those who don't cheat by reading last chapters first, what makes you keep reading to the end of a novel?

Suspense and cliff hangers help propel me through a story, but I don't want to dwell in those places of not knowing. What keeps me going is my desire to experience the ending. I want that sense of completion, that "aha!" moment, and the satisfaction of resolution or of confirming my suspicions. I don't like the no-man's land of not knowing.

I think this feature of story bears out in life, too. It is just that as actors in our own stories, we aren't privy to what comes next. We keep making decisions as we come to them without knowing exactly where our choices will take us in this long middle of our lives. Sometimes, we get the satisfaction of finishing a subplot, but in many other situations, we're stuck indefinitely not knowing.

Since there has been no objective test used to diagnose Parkinson's disease, I am stuck in a state of not knowing. The evidence all points to my having the disease, but no test can confirm the diagnosis. So when news about possible tests that can confirm a clinical Parkinson's diagnosis, I take notice. It is almost like getting news that the final sequel of a series will be released soon.

If Juliet Had Parkinson's
May 12, 2014

~~~~~~

I thought a bit of humor was in order today. My apologies to Shakespeare. Adapted from *Romeo and Juliet*, Act II, Scene II

JULIET:
O, dopamine[1], dopamine, wherefore art
   thou dopamine?
Deny thy absence and come to me
   again, Or if thou wilt not, a substitute I
   must accept,
I'll require a dopamine agonist.[2]
'Tis but thy absence that is my enemy.
Thou art thyself, though not my substan-
   tia nigra[3] (without thee),
What's substantia nigra? It controls
   hand, and foot,
And arm, and face, and any other part
Belonging to this woman. Oh, return to
   me again!
What's in thy presence? That which we
   ingest as dopamine[4]
Does not move my feet.
So agonists or levodopa serve, with
   friend carbidopa,
To take thy place. But thy absence is

---

1 Dopamine is a neurotransmitter in the brain that regulates movement and emotion. Having too little dopamine results in Parkinson's disease's symptoms.
2 Dopamine agonists are a class of drugs used to treat Parkinson's.
3 The part in the midbrain that produces dopamine.
4 Because it cannot cross the blood-brain barrier.

sore felt.
Dopamine, quit thy absence,
And with thy presence, which should be
a part of me, Move all myself.

CROSSING THE BRIDGE
July 1, 2014

~~~~~~

A couple of weeks ago, my husband and I returned from a trip to the state of Washington to celebrate our daughter's graduation from college. We drove there over the course of four days taking the northernmost U.S. route (Route 2) from the Upper Peninsula of Michigan all the way to Montana before dropping down to Interstate 90 to cross Washington.

The trip required traversing the Rocky and Cascade mountain ranges. I knew from our last trip that I did not want to drive through one of the highest mountain passes in Washington, so I agreed to drive across the plains of eastern Washington. My husband rested, promising to take over for me when we got into the foothills of the Cascades.

We were zipping along a sunny, flat expanse when the road started winding long before I expected it. Then the wind began gusting and whipping around though the sky was bright blue. Traffic forced me to clip along at a brisk pace, and we hurtled up and around a curve only to see the one thing worse than driving through a mountain pass in my book—a long, long, long bridge over the Columbia River.

I had forgotten about the bridge.

Since I was busy avoiding rappelling down a mountain in a mini-van rather than snapping photos, I didn't take a picture of this most terrifying feat of architecture, but I will not forget it. The winding, hilly road leading to the bridge gave us ample opportunity for sneak peeks of what was to come. By the time I realized our jeopardy, I had missed all of the pull-offs where I could have let my husband take over the driving. I was going to have to cross the bridge going around 70 miles per hour with a gusting cross wind capriciously trying to flip us into the Columbia River.

I thought that bridge would never end. I won't even attempt to convey the terror I felt in those few short moments of my life. Suffice it to say, I pulled off at the first possible spot once we made it to dry, solid land. Unlike that safe place, my face was not dry and my constitution was about as solid as a half-chilled Jell-O Jiggler.

For some reason this story came to mind as I was contemplating the fact that 2014 is now half over. How has 2014 gone for you so far? Are you zipping along through the plains of life? Or are you climbing a mountain or broken down on the side of the road?

Whatever the case, this halfway point is a good time to pull into a rest stop and consider how the journey is going. Here comes the rest of 2014, and ready or not, we're crossing that bridge.

When Life Gives You Garbanzo Beans
July 10, 2014

~~~~~~

My junior year of college, one of my college room-mates brought a case of canned food to our apart-ment to supplement our collective pantry. The kicker—the cans did not have labels. I don't remember where she procured the food, but I do remember the two ways to find out what was in each can—open it or decipher its stamped code. My roommate knew the codes, so as long as we asked her, we avoided pot-luck dinners.

I used to wish the paths of life had clear labels like products in the local supermarket. The array of life choices was overwhelming. As a budding perfectionist, I imagined only one route through life was correct for me, and I could find it if only I could decipher the clues. So I set out on a quest to "do" life as perfectly as possible by cracking its "codes."

Utilizing the experience of others whenever possible, I avoided unwanted waste and surprise when opening up life's cans, but I found that life often gives us encoded cans that no expertise or X-ray vision can penetrate. You simply have to open them up and figure out what to do with the contents.

Four decades into the journey, I'm a little better at accepting life's surprises. So instead of cherry pie, what would you say to a Deep Dish Garbanzo Bean Chocolate Chip Cookie?[1]

---

1 *(To prevent a heated discussion about life being au naturel—not frozen or canned—may I say all metaphors break down. I would bet my can opener on it.)*

An Honest-to-Goodness Day Job

July 26, 2014

After being gainfully unemployed for a little over a year, I finally landed a job—an honest-to-goodness, forty-hour-a-week, Monday-to-Friday, daylight-hour job as a technical writer. Last Friday, I came home, made supper, and sat in a stupor until stumbling up to bed before ten o'clock—on a Friday night. The first week on a job is taxing in more ways than the line items on the pay stub. After two weeks, I am still doing the Ben Franklin life hack—early to bed, early to rise—but my energy levels aren't nearly as low when I get home.

It is going to take time to adjust to my new schedule, but I have already come up with two beautiful things about this position (besides the paycheck)—evenings and weekends without work. When I leave this job, I leave. The work stays in the office. I don't have papers to grade or lesson plans to create as I did with teaching. It is truly a day job at least for now, and I am thankful for the opportunity.

A Travel Update
August 3, 2014

Trekking through the asteroid field of summer distractions and encounters with work of the full-time kind have limited my travel updates and left me pondering what will become of my blog, *A Path Not Chosen*.

Over the past year or so, this outpost in cyber space has gradually evolved into something quite different from its genesis—a place for me to write about my journey with Parkinson's disease. Now that I am well into the third year of living with Parkinson's, I find I don't have much to say about it. I am not cured and don't know everything there is to know about the disease, but writing about it has lost its appeal. Perhaps, part of the reason for this is that I am experiencing a respite from my worst symptoms based on a couple of changes I made this year.

Change One: A New Attitude toward Medication

In early 2014, I decided I couldn't tough it out without medication any longer. My tremor and muscle stiffness were beginning to affect my ability to do basic tasks like typing or relaxing my muscles enough to get to sleep at night. After trying a couple of medications that did not help or had terrible side effects, I decided I would change my attitude toward medication and consented to trying levodopa (with carbidopa).

I did not want to take this medication because everything I read indicated it should be the last resort for patients with young-onset Parkinson's disease. It can cause dyskenesia (involuntary muscle movements), and it seems to lose its efficacy at alleviating symptoms after using it for a number of years (though this could also be caused by the disease worsening over time). I decided to take the risk when the other alternative mentioned was Deep Brain Stimulation (DBS). I am not ready for brain surgery, despite the shift in thinking that DBS should be used earlier in the progression of the disease rather than later.

The medication has helped. When it is working, I have little to no tremor and my muscles relax and seem to work almost as well as they did pre-Parkinson's. Soon after I began taking the medication, the results of a study of levodopa came out that indicate it should be considered as an early treatment option. That helped me feel less anxious about my choice to take medication.

Change Two: A New Neurologist

The other change I made was to find a neurologist who specializes in neurological movement disorders like Parkinson's disease. After one appointment, I am convinced that it was a good move to make. He has helped me adjust the way I take my medication so that it works better, and he emphasizes other lifestyle choices that can help patients live well with Parkinson's.

After making these two changes, I feel almost normal again, and several people have commented that they've noticed the difference. I don't know how long this respite will last, but I am enjoying it while I can.

As for the fate of *A Path Not Chosen*, I don't think it will be going anywhere, but my captain's logs may be less frequent for the foreseeable future.

SETTLE DOWN!

May 5, 2014

~~~~~~

Settle down!
Sit quietly!
Be still and know...
If I can no longer be still, can I know?
Or does my body cry out when my mouth
   would not?

No movement = quiet.
No movement = stillness.
No movement = settled.

But I can't not move.
Not anymore.

Drugs bring moments of quiet to my
   body.
But not always.
Not continually.
Not reliably.

Just relax!
Chill!
Sit down and rest a while.

My muscles fire constantly.
Relax. Tense. Relax. Tense. Tense. Tense.
   Tense.
An ever-ready mouser with no prey.

Walking, moving, going somewhere,
It is in those actions that my body forgets

its contrariness.

Can quiet be found in motion?
Can stillness be found in motion?
Can I be settled in motion?
Will I ever be still—quiet—settled again?

Stuck on My Tuffet

November 30, 2014

~~~~~~

Little Miss Muffet
Sat on a tuffet
Eating her curds and whey.
Along came a spider
Who sat down beside her
And frightened Miss Muffet away.

Today was the first Sunday of Advent, and today's sermon focused on fear. That was especially appropriate for me, as three years ago today, one of those big, hairy, eight-legged fears we all dread came and sat down beside me—yes, it is anniversary number three.

Like Miss Muffet, I prefer to run from big, hairy, eight-legged fears, but unlike her, I couldn't run away from the source of this one. It has lodged itself permanently in my brain. I have been stuck on my tuffet with this nasty little spider of a disease quietly spinning its web of destruction around and within me.

During this triennium, I have done my share of fighting the fears that accompany a chronic disease, but as I contemplated the third anniversary of my diagnosis, I realized that lately I have been trying to flee the fears by looking the other way and ignoring their presence through denial or keeping busy since I can't physically escape the source of my fears. When I am forced to turn back around and see the menacing, hairy legs of my future, debilitating fears wash over me once again, and like so many who have come before me, I need to hear this choice again—"Do not be afraid."

"But how?" I ask.

So far, I have no definitive answer aside from the image of a giant straight razor shaving the hairy spider legs of my future.

Choices on a Path Not Chosen

The Fourth Year

〜〜〜

The Scarecrow sat in the big throne and the others stood respectfully before him....“We are not so unlucky,” said the new ruler, “for this Palace and the Emerald City belong to us, and we can do just as we please. When I remember that a short time ago I was up on a pole in a farmer's cornfield, and that now I am the ruler of this beautiful City, I am quite satisfied with my lot.... If Dorothy would only be contented to live in the Emerald City,” continued the Scarecrow, “we might all be happy together.”
~L. Frank Baum, *The Wonderful Wizard of Oz*

When 2015 arrived, medications had allowed me to live almost normally for most of the previous year, keeping the most noticeable symptoms at bay. Some days I could almost forget I had Parkinson's. But like Dorothy, I still had obstacles that would test my ability to be content on my path not chosen—I still wanted to go home.

When a Day Is Like a Week of Sleepless Nights

March 1, 2015

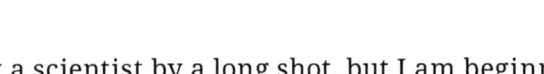

I am not a scientist by a long shot, but I am beginning to believe that the length of a day can vary person to person. Why have I developed this hypothesis?

Insomnia.

I have struggled with this off and on since I began taking medications for Parkinson's, but it has been especially troublesome since last fall. Back in December, I went most of a work week with an accumulated total of eleven hours of rest. And yes, I said rest, not sleep, because though I was exhausted and did the bedtime routine hack, during that one long "day" I never felt like I actually had restorative sleep.

Couple this with a series of sleep-disrupting events including a bout with a virus before and after the holidays, a two-week emergency trip to Singapore (another story) complete with jet lag on either end, and a full-time job, and the following sleep schedule becomes the norm:

- Go to bed no later than 10:00. Sleep 4 hours.
- Go to bed no later than 10:00. Sleep 5-6 hours.
- Go to bed at 7:00. Sleep 10 hours.
- Take a nap if a short-night cycle happens to fall on a weekend.

Yes, I am investigating the usual suspects like caffeine, lack of a regular sleep schedule, too much screen time in the evening, too little sunlight and exercise in the day (thanks to frigid temps), and timing of my Parkinson's medications. Yet thinking too much about it and struggling to go to sleep do not help.

The short nights are burdensome and wearying, but oh how much sweeter are the mornings when you awake after an uninterrupted night of seven or more hours of sleep. Thankfully, I am about due for a long night of sleep in this new world where a week can be as one long day.

No Synchronicity

March 5, 2015

The waves beckon,
I answer,
Making my nightly trek into the drink
Doggedly pushing through water
Breaking itself against the land
To that quiet place beyond the chaos
Where an abandoned vessel
(As seaworthy as a wooden shoe)
Bobs on the glassy tresses of the sea..

I clamber in, lie down, and wait
Rocking gently to a place dubbed Nod,
But far below deep calls to deep.
The echoes agitate the calm.
My frozen stare drills dark above.
Unable to move or shut my eyes,
Soon I am tossed into the waters,
Fighting, thrashing against the tempest
Trying to beat it to submission.

Peace.
That is all I want.

Rest.
That is all I need.

Exhaustion.
Can it get me there?

Limp.

Still.

I do a dead man's float,
Shielding my eyes from the first speckle
    of sunrise.
If I can only catch the right wave,
Perhaps, I will end up where I want to be.

But tonight.

.no synchronicity.

I slap.

   Off.

.Beat.

Against the surge.

Only to find myself beached.
At sunrise.
Unable to chase the retreating tide
With skittering terns.

What's Inside?

April 2, 2015

～～～

As a child and teenager sifting through the box of possibilities for my future, I recall at least three things I did not want to do—

- Study English
- Teach, or
- Work for a large corporation.

I have now done all three.

As I was raising my children, I remember one thing I wanted to do once they grew up—go back to work full time and pursue a legitimate career with legitimate defined as a meaningful job with a living salary.

When I landed a job as a full-time technical writer last summer, I had the opportunity to fulfill that "to do" on my list, but I also ended up doing one of the "not to dos"—work for a large corporation. In the end, I have found my fears about working for "the man" to be largely unfounded and grew to enjoy working with those in my department.

Change is in the air, however, and I have stepped down from my full-time technical writing position.

Like I told my coworkers, the choice to resign was brought about by several factors, but the biggest one stems from the fact that I am living with Parkinson's disease.

It is not that I am physically incapable of working. On the contrary, the medications I started taking in the spring of 2014 have given me a new lease on life. During the day, when the medication is working, I almost feel normal again.

- My tremor disappears.
- My muscle stiffness goes away, including the uncomfortable cramping and curling of the muscles in my left foot.
- I swing my left arm without thinking about it.
- My overall mood improves.

In fact, I didn't share my Parkinson's challenge with my coworkers until I made the choice to leave because it did not affect my ability to do my job. (My neurologist backed me up on my choice not to share in that context.) But during the last few months, insomnia has wreaked havoc with my sleep schedule and energy level. I have found I can get through an eight-hour day, but once I am home, I often have had nothing left. The phrase "I gave at the office," takes on a different meaning when you have little energy to give to the rest of your life.

So despite the many reasons why I felt I should keep the job, I chose to leave. As long as I feel well physically (other than the exhaustion), I want to spend the resources I have on other endeavors. It's time for me to revisit my box of possibilities and see what is inside.

Yes, You Do Have Choices on a Path Not Chosen

May 3, 2015

〜〜〜

How many choices do you think you make each day? Ten, a hundred, a thousand? When the idea for this post popped into my head, I thought I would call it "A Thousand Choices." That seemed high until I began to think of all of the choices I have already made today:

- Ignore the song birds at 4:30 a.m.
- Bury my head under my pillow and try to go back to sleep.
- Begin to give into the inevitability of the day when the sun arrives.
- Try desperately to go back to dreamland and finish that dream.
- Ignore the sounds of my son making coffee in the kitchen.
- Lie there for a few more minutes.
- Refuse to open my eyes.
- Decide it is useless to stay in bed.
- Stretch my legs.
- Wiggle my toes.
- Think about getting up to run.
- Notice the tightness in my leg muscles, and remember that I had a tough work out about 12 hours earlier.
- Decide to exercise later in the day.
- Open my eyes, one by one.
- Shield my eyes against the glare of the sun.

- Reach over and pick up my phone to avoid getting out of bed a few more minutes.

That was all before I got out of bed. And I know I missed some micro-decisions along the way. It is mind-boggling to stop and count all of the decisions we make. In fact, it is downright tiring. This is why we automate so many things in our lives. We create habits and routines so that we don't have to think about the millions of decisions we must make every day.

So far, I haven't experienced the Parkinson's symptom where I freeze, unable to connect my decision with my body's response, but it may happen someday. Something that I have experienced, however, is feeling like I don't have choices. In an effort to battle this feeling, I have learned to remind myself, "But you do."

I may dislike all or most of the options, but it is generally a lie to say, "I don't have a choice." Almost every situation—even the most terrible ones—give you at least have two options.

- Yes/no
- Do/don't
- Speak/stay silent
- Laugh/cry
- To be/not to be
- This/that

Sometimes one choice is clearly better than the other, and other times, it is a wash—they're equally good or bad.

Once we choose, then we can say, "I don't have to make that choice again," but we can rarely say, "I didn't have a choice." We make choices all day long whether we think about it or not.

You may find yourself somewhere you don't want to be. You may find you can never return to what once was. Yet, you still have choices even if you're a few shy of a million options.

Letting Your Life Speak

April 7, 2015

~~~~~~~

Listen to your life. See it for the fathomless mystery it is.
In the boredom and pain of it, no less than in the excite-
ment and gladness: touch, taste, smell your way to the
holy and hidden heart of it, because in the last analysis
all moments are key moments, and life itself is grace.
~Frederick Buechner[1]

S top a moment. Pull out the ear buds. Take your hand off the mouse. Put down your beverage of choice. Now, close your eyes and listen for a moment or two.

Do you hear it?

Do you hear what your life is saying to you?

I don't know about you, but for me, listening requires intentionality. And when it comes to listening to my life, sometimes I wonder if I need hearing aids. The noise of busyness and obligations drowns out the even, quiet tones of life, and if we're not careful, we'll arrive at the other end of our journey full of regret and without a clue about what life said to us along the way.

Life sometimes installs speed bumps that force us to slow down and pay attention. Health crises, job changes, deaths, moves, relationship changes, and other life-redirecting events require us to discard the trivial and strip down to the core of who we are and what life is. I have

---

1 Buechner, Frederick. *Now and Then: A Memoir of Vocation.* Harper Collins, New York, 1983.

experienced a couple of these already in 2015, and I am trying to listen better than I have in the past.

But it is not easy.

It has been a week since I stepped down from my position as a technical writer. I have had people ask what I am doing now that I am not working at a J-O-B. Depending on who asks, I mumble one of the stock answers I have come up with about rest or housework or looking into potential part-time or telecommuting opportunities.

I have been doing all of these things. But I have also been reading and researching and praying about my next steps. Reading *The Art of Work* by Jeff Goins reminded me of the Frederick Buechner quote at the beginning of this post. After referring to Buechner's call to "listen to our lives," Goins follows up with this:

> *What Buechner was saying is that awareness doesn't just happen; it must be cultivated. If you pay attention to your life and the lessons it can teach you, you won't feel so lost. Your story will seem less like a series of disjointed events and more like a beautifully complex narrative unfolding before you. You will understand each setback, inconvenience, and frustration as something more than what it appears to be. And perhaps, as you listen to it, your life will speak.[1]*

In many ways, I feel that I have been listening though I know I can listen better.

- **Listening.** It is what I have done the first four years living with Parkinson's, trying to make sense of this permanent detour in my life.

---

1 Goins, Jeff. *The Art of Work.* Nelson Books: Nashville, 2015

- **Listening.** It is what I am trying to do with the rest of the time I have been given.
- **Listening.** It is a place where I have gotten stuck in the past because I didn't like what I heard or didn't act on what I did hear.

So the question I ask myself each day is whether I am willing to act and let my life speak?

- **Speaking.** It is sharing in the journey of others, swapping travel notes, and uncovering life's moments of grace.
- **Speaking.** It is accepting what we cannot change and making the changes we can.
- **Speaking.** It is standing up and walking down a path we have not chosen despite the challenges we are sure to encounter.

Do I Still Want to Go "Home"?

Into the Future

~~~~~~~

"Your Silver Shoes will carry you over the desert," replied Glinda. *"If you had known their power you could have gone back to your Aunt Em the very first day you came to this country."*
~L. Frank Baum, *The Wonderful Wizard of Oz*

F iction is unsatisfying when a story resolves in such a way that the hero's journey never had to take place. It seems like the "good" witches played a cruel joke on Dorothy by not telling her that the witch's shoes she wore throughout her time in Oz had the power to take her back to her family all along.

The Scarecrow, the Tin Man, and the Cowardly Lion point out that without Dorothy, they would never have gotten their greatest desires—a brain, a heart, and courage. Though this observation doesn't eliminate the sting of having been played, Dorothy is glad to have known and helped her companions.

In addition to the friendships, Dorothy's journey through Oz gave her experiences that caused her to grow and change. Would she have been as thankful if she had returned home immediately?

Contrived ending or not, Dorothy finally gets to go home, and when she does, Baum quickly wraps up the story in a handful of sentences:

> ...just before her was the new farmhouse Uncle Henry built after the cyclone had carried away the old one. Uncle Henry was milking the cows in the barnyard, and Toto had jumped out of her arms and was running toward the barn, barking furiously.
>
> Dorothy stood up and found she was in her stocking-feet. For the Silver Shoes had fallen off in her flight through the air, and were lost forever in the desert
>
> Aunt Em had just come out of the house to water the cabbages when she looked up and saw Dorothy running toward her.
>
> "My darling child!" she cried, folding the little girl in her arms and covering her face with kisses. "Where in the world did you come from?"
>
> "From the Land of Oz," said Dorothy gravely. "And here is Toto, too. And oh, Aunt Em! I am so glad to be at home again!"

In the original story, the house actually blew away, and the whole adventure was not simply a dream as it was portrayed in the movie. Aunt Em and Uncle Henry apparently thought Dorothy died in the cyclone, so the ending in the book feels quite abrupt and anti-climactic.

Yet, it provides insight into how we deal with the unchosen paths we find ourselves on in life, and how they affect our deepest longings. It is telling that Glinda says the magic shoes could have taken her back to her Aunt Em, rather than saying they could have taken her *home.* Dorothy got her wish to return to the place she called home, but it was not the home she had left. Her home had changed physically due to the cyclone and emotionally because of her family's need to adapt to her disappearance and apparent death. Dorothy also changed on her journey through Oz. We like to think of "home" as a place of permanence and stability, yet it changes as surely as everything else in this temporal world.

In a paradoxical way, my first four years with Parkinson's disease have brought me back to the "home" I longed for—a place of relative health both physically and mentally. No, I haven't been cured, but by taking on the challenges of this path not chosen, I am stronger and fitter due to changes in diet and exercise. Learning how to get the best results from the medications I take, has given me the ability to function almost normally most days. My tremor disappears and my muscles behave.

The physical changes have contributed to better mental health as well. While the spectre of depression never disappears, I know what I need to do to keep it at bay, and I try to take those steps before its gray fog overcomes me.

I didn't realize what I had until it was taken away. I was unaware of the gifts of life and health and how I had become blind to the colors of life. As I begin my fifth year living with Parkinson's, I have had to ask whether I really want to go back to the version of "home" I had prior to my diagnosis.

When I am honest, I say absolutely not.

While I wish I could have learned what I know now without having Parkinson's and I don't look forward to the further obstacles and hardships that will come as I continue on my journey, I am thankful this experience has helped make me a healthier person despite having a chronic, incurable disease.

Will I still have this perspective as the disease progresses? It is hard to know. When this journey began, I feared being an invalid five years down the road, but I am not. Advances and discoveries continue to unlock the mysteries of Parkinson's giving hope that in the near future we'll know how to prevent, slow down, or even reverse the disease.

Whether or not that happens during my lifetime does not concern and consume me as it once might have. I know, however, that I may forget what I've learned when the way gets rough. I have kept these notes and share them with you, to remind us of these simple yet powerful truths:

> *We should be aware of and thankful for all we have—before we lose it.*

> *Life's in Technicolor—if we have the eyes to see it.*

> *And we always have choices—even on a path not chosen.*

WHAT IS PARKINSON'S DISEASE?

A Brief Introduction

~~~~~

When my current neurologist tells a patient he or she has Parkinson's disease he says, "The bad news is—you have Parkinson's. But the good news is—you have Parkinson's." For those unfamiliar with Parkinson's, here's a brief overview of the disease—the bad, the good, and the hopeful.

THE BAD NEWS

- Parkinson's is an incurable, neurodegenerative disorder of the brain that affects movement. Symptoms are caused by the death of neurons in the substantia nigra region of the brain, which is responsible for producing the neurotransmitter dopamine. Dopamine helps the body control movement. Once symptoms are noticeable it is estimated that between 60-80 percent of the neurons necessary to produce dopamine are dead or malfunctioning.
- Statistics vary, but it is estimated that one million people have Parkinson's in the U.S. alone.

Worldwide, the number grows to 7-10 million.[1] Because of the difficulty of diagnosis and the variety of ways Parkinson's manifests in individuals, many may go undiagnosed.

- According to the National Parkinson's Foundation, 62 is the average age for being diagnosed with Parkinson's, and those diagnosed under the age of 50 are considered to have young-onset Parkinson's disease.[2]

- Symptoms vary from person to person, but the primary motor symptoms often include resting tremors, muscle stiffness or spasticity, shuffling gait when walking, lack of arm swinging, freezing (the inability to move), reduced facial expression, difficulty swallowing, and a soft voice. Non-motor symptoms may include hyposmia (reduced sense of smell), depression, dementia, sleep disorders, drooling, and constipation.

THE GOOD NEWS

- It is one of the less aggressive neurological diseases, and it is not fatal, although complications associated with Parkinson's may eventually lead to death.

- The disease progresses slowly over years or even decades, and the progression is generally slower for young-onset patients.[3]

- Medications can help control the symptoms allowing many Parkinson's patients to lead a productive and full life.

---

1 "Statistics on Parkinson's." *Parkinson's Disease Foundation.* 2016. Web.
2 "Young-Onset Parkinson's?" *National Parkinson Foundation.* 2016. Web.
3 "What Is Parkinson's?" *National Parkinson Foundation.* 2016. Web.

- Deep brain stimulation, which has been compared to a pacemaker for the brain, applies controlled electrical impulses to the area of the brain controlling movement, and has been successful at significantly reducing symptoms in Parkinson's patients.
- Lifestyle choices such as exercising, getting sufficient sleep, reducing stress, and eating a healthy diet can alleviate some symptoms.

The Hopeful

Research efforts continue to explore and unravel the mystery of Parkinson's in order to provide better therapies and eventually a cure. To learn more about Parkinson's research, visit the following websites:

American Parkinson Disease Association
http://www.apdaparkinson.org

Michael J. Fox Foundation for Parkinson's Research
http://www.michaeljfox.org

National Parkinson Foundation
http://www.parkinson.org

Parkinson's Disease Foundation
http://www.pdf.org

About the Author

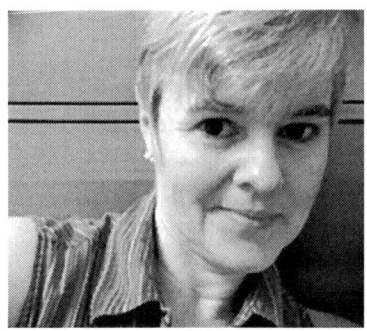

Sherri Tobias is a writer and educator. She has published a collection of short fiction, *Refractions*, in addition to blogging and writing articles. Several "heartbreaking works of staggering genius" await release from the prison of her mind in the near future.

If you ask Sherri where she's from, she may say she's homeless or home-full, having lived in or visited over twenty countries in which she resided in an unknown number of houses, huts, apartments, campers, and tents. She currently lives in Ohio with her family. You can find out more about Sherri on her website, **sherritobias.com**.

Fiction by Sherri Tobias

*What do you do when life sends you
in a direction you never wanted to go?*

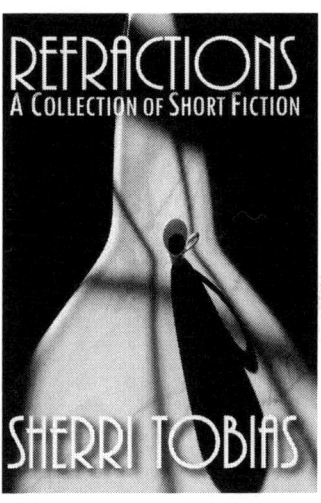

Each of the vignettes in *Refractions: A Collection of Short Fiction* explores challenges in the lives of three women and how new possibilities emerge from the ordinary stuff of life. The collection includes:

- **Liquid.** A new mother living in a new town wonders if she will ever regain the sense of belonging she had as a child while battling what she dubs "The Buckeye Blues."
- **Dandelions Dance.** A sidelined professional dancer, now a housewife and mother of a preschooler, struggles with her inability to pursue her passion.
- **The Fall.** A young detective investigating a suspicious death discovers his former kindergarten teacher, now homeless, will do almost anything to avoid the fall.

33155703R00093

Made in the USA
Middletown, DE
02 July 2016